AF441809

SPEAKING OF SEX

SPEAKING OF SEX:
Mothers and Daughters

Carol Kleiman
and
Catharine E. Kleiman

Bonus Books, Chicago

91   90   89   88   87   5   4   3   2   1

Library of Congress Catalog Card Number: 87-70663

International Standard Book Number: 0-933893-35-3

Bonus Books, Inc.
160 East Illinois Street
Chicago, Illinois 60611

Printed in the United States of America

To mutual and much-loved friends of this fortunate Mother–Daughter team: Marilyn Norehad, Ilana Diamond Rovner and Gayle Wilder

And to all Mothers and Daughters—and open communication

CONTENTS

INTRODUCTION

CAROL | Talking about *all* the "Facts of Life"—birth, love, sex, marriage, divorce, death—is difficult, I've found, often painful. Especially about sex. Especially with my daughter.

No wonder so many mothers avoid it!

But who is there better to deliver the message? When mothers talk, they are educating. Daughters absorb, perhaps to forget or reject later, but still, they listen. Talking about sex, one of the most vulnerable, complicated and wonderful aspects of human life, is a rare opportunity for sharing our own deep feelings and attitudes, to influence, to guide.

Talking about sex, however, cannot be taken out of context. It has to be part of your whole relationship with your daughter. My daughter and I do battle constantly. You should have heard us working on this book—maybe you did! But we are very close. And I am proud of that. We've worked at closeness all our lives.

Because of what we share, I have to admit I get very upset at the books that condemn all mothers in one fell swoop.

Christina Crawford's *Mommie Dearest* helps solidify the picture of mothers as monsters; and, in fact, its title takes a very sweet appellation—"Mommie," as in, "Mommie, get me a glass of water"—and turns it into a slur. Nancy Friday does the same in *My Mother/My Self*. Friday takes an especially hard swipe at daughters discussing sex with their mothers, who, she implies, are only waiting to swoop down on their daughters and terrorize and paralyze their sexuality. Another book along these painful lines is *My Mother's Keeper*, by B.D. Hyman, daughter of actress Bette Davis. "I am still recovering from the fact that a child of mine would write about me behind my back," Davis says in an open letter to her daughter in Davis' book, *This 'n That*.

Not all mothers are wonderful. Neither are all daughters. Occasionally, there is no hope to work out a relationship. But that is precisely what is necessary before sex can be something you discuss naturally, like grades, friends, careers. When it does work, it's a special gift for a mother and daughter.

Much popular writing—and good old Sigmund Freud —debases women, especially that eternal target, Mom. But the women's movement tells us all women count, an idea much more pleasing to me. "If I am to see myself and all women in this new way, if I am to love myself—love women—what about my Mother?" asks Judith Arcana in her book, *Our Mothers' Daughters*, which illuminates, probes and affirms mother–daughter relationships.

I love and respect Cathy. I want to protect her. I don't want her hurt. She is "my best piece of poetry," as Ben Jonson wrote about his child. So are my sons, Robert and Raymond. I want Cathy to have a full, rich life, with sex as a satisfying, sharing, exhilarating experience. There's only so much I can say. She must do her own thing, as she would put it.

The closeness and the distance are both integral parts of my relationship with Cathy: I would die for my daughter, but I would not live for her.

CATHY | Being close with your mother sounds good, but it's not easy to achieve. In fact, I think it's pretty rare. I feel lucky.

The doorway to intimacy is trust. And the only way you can ever establish trust is through open communication. Communication means talking, saying how you really feel about things—and this goes both ways. It's the mutual rapport between mother and daughter that creates a relationship.

Mother–daughter relationships are special. Each of you is undeniably a part of each other. Other friendships lack the built-in bond that mothers and daughters share. Ideally, each of you will cultivate that bond.

If you start with communication and openness, you not only have the beginnings of a good relationship with your mother, you also have the ingredients you will need to have good relationships with other people in your life. What a nice way to learn: in protective custody!

Many of the things that have bothered me growing up don't seem so overwhelming after talking them over with my mother. She's gone through so many of them herself. She's lived through a lot and that means, to me, that I can, too.

You can't get away from biology, and mothers and daughters have compelling biological similarities, even if they don't have the same minds or the same philosophies. Our shared femaleness is the constant, the basis for wanting to communicate. The differences are our own individual personalities, characters and emotions.

I like to think of myself as strong, independent—like my mother. However, as I reflect from my mother, I know myself. It's the old story of learning more by comparisons.

Here's how I view mother–daughter relationships: My mother's role is to share; mine is to learn, listen and compare. (Although I must admit in recent years I've started to give my mother a lot of advice!) I don't feel I have to adapt to everything she suggests or adhere to all she believes. But it is important to know what she believes. And I do. I know how my mother feels about many things, not just sex.

I keep stressing "open communication." I mean honesty. It doesn't work when mothers turn their talks into sermons or rigid guidelines of "This Is The Way It Is—Or

Else!" There is no communication when your mother talks at you and not with you. It is a fine line, but a critical one.

As much as I believe in a close relationship, there are still a lot of times and many things I do not want to talk to my mother about. But that's okay. It's normal. In many of those situations, I'm much more comfortable talking to my friends.

And one important lesson I've learned is you also have to rely on yourself and your own experiences. You don't have to seek advice on everything, especially those things you feel in your gut, the things you know are right for you.

As close as we are, some things are too private, too embarrassing, too touchy to talk about with my mother. That's when I go to my friends. They have a different perspective: They're not so worried about protecting me. Mothers spend a lifetime doing that for their daughters. It's hard to get them to stop.

In working on this book with my mother, I've discovered a lot of things have happened in my life that I don't remember, especially between my mother and me. Or, my version of what happened is radically different from hers.

The most important thing, though, is that I have always felt I *could* talk to my mother, that I could go to her and say anything. I have friends who wouldn't dare talk to their moms about anything. But I can. It is my choice, when I want to. She is a security I can rely on.

When you have a good relationship with your mother,

you're lucky, because you really have some place to turn to, someone to talk to, someone who cares.

And best of all, someone you love and who loves you.

Carol Kleiman

Cathy Kleiman

LET'S TALK ABOUT THE STORK

MOTHER | When I was a little girl, I played with dolls, like most girl children of my pre-Barbie generation. And, like most little girls in the days before both sexes were offered both dolls and trucks to play with—a far more enlightening choice—I fantasized I was the Mother and the doll (I remember my Shirley Temple doll the best) was the Baby.

But there all similarities to my other friends end: The little girls in my neighborhood cooed over their dolls with terms of endearment and imitated their mothers by giving orders to their dolls. Not me. I always had serious conversations with my dolls.

I loved my Shirley Temple doll deeply but I never used baby talk. I never cooed—though I must admit I did a lot of that with my own babies. I never chastized about how naughty she was, though I certainly heard it often enough myself. Instead, I talked in a straightforward manner about things on my mind, hoping to find answers in the process.

I must have been a rare sight, the time I wept real tears, which my doll could not do, about not being allowed on the neighborhood football team. I was not then smart enough to be angry about being left out because I was a girl. I was mad because it was *my* football!

I talked sincerely to my doll about things I wondered about, such as where do babies come from and how did they get there in the first place? I could not get satisfactory answers from my own mother who, when forced to answer, would implicate the stork. The frustration of not knowing and having a vague feeling of being laughed at was mitigated somewhat by what today would probably be called "doll therapy." I did get comfort from talking to my doll, even though I got no answers from her, either.

Eventually, I got too old for dolls. I reluctantly gave them up at age eleven, long after my friends had, because my doll was my confidante. How nice for me if my confidante had been my mother. Unfortunately, even at that great age I still knew nothing about sex, or life or death. And still, I couldn't get any answers.

My mother, born early in the century, was simply constitutionally unable to talk about anything relating to S-E-X. Also, I was very late in developing, so she probably saw no immediate urgency to confront the issue.

In addition to her Victorian approach, a long and hard

struggle for survival had also made her mute on this threatening subject. I was a post-Depression baby, and my mother often told me, "You're lucky to have been born." I always wondered, sometimes humorously, what she meant by that, but she would not elaborate.

And that is how I grew up believing absolutely in the stork, despite all evidence in my fecund neighborhood to the contrary. I was the youngest, so I never saw my mother pregnant. Even if I had, I was so naive I fear I might have believed then that babies were brought by the hospital.

How my state of innocence was maintained for so long is hard for me to understand. I had two older sisters and many close friends. I read seven books a week—the limit I could borrow from the library—but it never occurred to me to read one on sex. I did well in school. And yet, I knew nothing about sexual intercourse or even what menstruation meant until I was fourteen years old. I had no idea there was such a thing as an orgasm until I was nineteen.

It's embarrassing to relate these facts, but they are true: As a child, I was sexually-deprived of facts.

I remember me at twelve, flat-chested and wearing undershirts. My friends had long ago discarded their long-awaited training bras—I always wondered for what they were training—for the real thing. One hot summer night, wearing the kind of T-shirt later made popular by Marlon Brando (who filled it out better than I did) and in my red Jantzen shorts, I paraded in front of my parents and some guests, demanding to know The Truth.

"Mother, Mother!" I whined. "Tell me, *please*, where do babies come from?"

"Well, dear," she said mildly, half-smiling, half-embarrassed in front of her friends, "the stork brings babies to married women."

It was the first time she had given me additional information about the stork and its predilection for wedded females only. Her friends nodded in agreement and I leaped on it with what I thought was admirable quickness.

"But Mother," I crowed triumphantly, thinking I'd caught her at last, "how does the stork know who's married?"

I had her, but a lot of good it did me. I still got no answers, no explanations. No one gave me an illustrated book to read, no teacher mentioned sex in school, so I continued knowing nothing. It's no coincidence I was also the last kid on my block to learn there was no Santa Claus.

My state of stupidity ended at age sixteen, when my friend Jack told me about the role menstruation plays in procreation and what women and men do to make babies. I was lucky—he told me gently, without embarrassment. He had grown up with the facts and was comfortable with them.

What he thought of my questions, I don't know. But I didn't let on I was asking out of ignorance: I pretended I already knew everything, that I was asking for a friend. Unfortunately, he delicately omitted the subject of orgasm, so that wasn't added to my store of knowledge for a few more years.

Because of my protracted naivety, it was only by dumb luck alone that I didn't get into serious, life-damaging trouble before then. Because of the furtiveness that surrounded the subject in my house, with the unspoken message that sex was something very dirty and bad, it's also fortunate that today I have such a positive attitude about sex. I think it's fun!

When I finally learned my biology and later, my sexuality, I determined no daughter of mine would ever be so ignorant. To tell the truth, when I learned the truth, I felt ridiculous, betrayed. What hadn't I known all along?

For years, I cringed when I thought about that little girl in the T-shirt on that hot summer night. I had thought I was so smart and in reality I was so dumb! Today, I look back on that scene with nostalgia, but I wouldn't want it ever to be repeated, certainly not in my house or by me.

Jack was a wonderful friend, but he wasn't the best person to teach me the facts of life. I needed a female person to talk things over with, to explain the mysteries and the emotions.

I had other barriers to learning the facts of life: I had no brothers, and my father's body was always carefully hidden from his daughters, so even when I began to learn that ovum and sperm meet, I was not quite sure of the equipment involved in such a transaction.

Because in my house we never spoke about sex or the different "plumbing" of the two sexes, I also had no socially-acceptable words, no vocabulary for body parts or for the sexual act itself. That made me self-conscious about talking about sex and also stalled the learning process for me. My friends, when I finally understood what they had been talking about all along, spoke easily, using street words, slang or euphemisms for vaginas, penises, urination and the like.

I didn't like those words, which I felt were demeaning, but even so, I went along with the crowd. I was so relieved to know what they were talking about—at last!

Once again, I vowed *my* daughter would learn the parts of her body and everything else she needed to know to be in charge of her body.

At the same time, I vowed I would tell my daughter—and my sons—in real words, not scientific polysyllables but words with respect for the functions described.

No baby talk when talking about babies. And no shame, either. I kept my promise: I never used baby talk at all with Cathy. That's probably one of the reasons she's so articulate today.

As you can see, I had a lot of incentive to talk frankly about sex with my daughter. I also had a lot of reason to find it difficult to do so, but I refused to be stymied. Not all mothers see the urgent need to be upfront. I wish they did. Talking about sex is an essential communication, especially when it comes from a loved one.

So I started early and spoke clearly.

I tried to make Cathy feel comfortable about her body from birth, something I had to teach myself to do. I taught her that nothing connected with the body is "dirty." When she was very little, I did not stand up and give authoritative lectures on sex, but I do think I helped create the idea in her that sex is a wonderful invention, to be enjoyed in a responsible way.

I wanted my daughter always to know that sex is a part

of life, not to be hidden, not to be snickered at. I wanted her to know it's a very personal relationship, something positive—even before she had all the facts in place. That's the kind of groundwork I believe absolutely necessary, even before our daughters learn the exact anatomical details. A healthy attitude—which is most easily shared by mothers who have one to share—is a precursor to confidence for making responsible decisions.

That type of education cannot be left for the time when hormones begin to rage. It could be too late then.

Ironically, the specter of the AIDS epidemic provides a good opportunity to make up for lost time. Mothers who previously have felt too uncomfortable to speak about sex with their daughters now have a compelling reason to do so. The necessity to discuss how to prevent this dreaded disease overrides some mothers' embarrassment about talking about sexual matters with daughters. Now, they know they must: It's a matter of life or death. And daughters who don't want to discuss "intimate" matters with their mothers will now listen, too. And for the same reason: Life or death. After pouring out your fears about AIDS and having a dialogue with your daughter about precautionary measures, Mothers will find the rest of the conversation much easier. The AIDS epidemic will permit some mothers to make up for years of silence—a rare example of good coming out of evil!

I had grown up knowing nothing about sex, not a word. Not even when I finally got my period. Knowing how painful ignorance is, I was determined to tell my daughter from Day One everything I knew about sex.

This communication-utopia was my dream. It isn't necessarily my daughter's. She didn't always want to listen and she didn't always want to know everything. Even as a child, Cathy determined the parameters of our discussions. And she hasn't changed. Recently, when I started to tell her about a sexual escapade of a mutual acquaintance, she stopped me, saying, "Oh, Mother, I don't want to hear about that!" Which only goes to prove the world is round: As a daughter, I would have given anything to have my mother talk to me so easily about sex.

I know many mothers and daughters who are closeasthis, but they never talk about sex, not out of mutual respect for privacy but out of fear. Fear of rejection. I think that's a shame.

When you want to be close with someone, it's hard to close down a certain percentage of your life and leave it out. It's bound to affect the relationship and lead to lies, duplicity and cover-ups.

"Oh, please don't tell my mother!" one of Cathy's friends begged me after talking to Cathy in front of me about her very close relationship with her boyfriend.

She was very young, only fifteen, and she needed an adult to talk to, someone responsible for her, someone who loved her. She didn't need me, Cathy's mother, though I tried to help. She needed her mother.

I'm not a scientist, sociologist, sexologist, gynecologist or theologian. I'm a journalist. My daughter is a college student. We certainly do not qualify as experts on sex. But we do know how to discuss all things close to our hearts with one another. We learned to trust each other enough to share intimacies.

How we reached that mutually-satisfying state in life may not work for everyone or anyone else. But we did it —without having any of the credentials noted above—and I hope that inspires others to try. I had to give it a try, because I didn't want my daughter ever to go through what I had gone through.

Happily, it worked for us.

DAUGHTER | I always felt badly when my mom told me how she never had anyone to talk to when she was growing up. I've never had that problem, but that still doesn't mean it is always easy talking to my mother about everything. After all, she's still my mother, and most daughters don't want to be put in a position where they think they'll be judged.

And the subject of sex is *really* volatile. Yet, if you've grown up talking with your mother about it, the way I have, it feels unnatural NOT to. I don't remember the early lessons but I do remember the message: My mom is someone I can confide in. My mom will answer all questions. She is always there for me if I need her.

Unfortunately, storks were still popular when I was a little girl and probably still are today. My friends often talked about how their mothers had "found" a baby one lovely day, either on the doorstep or in the bedroom.

Not only did I just miss being part of the Baby Boom, I

also missed the anatomically "correct" dolls—though I haven't seen them and cannot testify to whether they actually are fully "correct" or what they teach the children who play with them. I never noticed that my Barbie doll had a real "female" chest, which was so shocking to many of my mother's generation.

What I do know is that if my mother hadn't taught me about sex, it would have been almost as hard for me to learn about it as it was for her. I'd have few places to go to get honest answers. I grew up knowing—and it stood me in good stead—that sex is not anything shameful or anything to be embarrassed about. Just private.

Despite my own experience, I understand why some daughters cannot talk to their mothers about sex. I can see generational hangups that would make it hard to talk to your mother. If your mother never offered you information when you were very young, it might be hard to be the one to bring up the subject—especially when you already know sex is something "unmentionable."

Later, in adolescence, it might seem to you "uncool" to be close to your mother. And, if you're in a rebellious stage, which usually coincides with adolescence, you often don't feel like talking about personal things with your mother. Especially if it's something you feel very sensitive about. During my rebellious stage, the communication I had with my mother consisted mostly of my stubbornly saying, "No!"

Also, it would be very difficult to discuss sex with your mother if she has laid down a strict code, rigid rules about sex or seemingly inflexible emotions about it. What if you have questions you know she wouldn't approve of? I don't think I'd be able to approach my mother if she projected a negative attitude.

In high school, I had a friend from a strict religious family that blatantly let her know sex before marriage is a sin. When she did get involved with a guy, she was torn between emotions for him and the constant threats she had heard her whole life and continued to hear from her parents.

That made it impossible to talk to them. She needed to know about birth control. She was in love for the first time and would have loved to talk to her mom about being in love and how wonderful it was. But she couldn't. It was a shame. Religion, morals and built-in values that were inflexible made it impossible for her mother to listen to her, even to hear her. Her mom's way of showing love was to warn her about what she thought was evil. When her daughter fell in love, her mom only increased her warnings, rather than confront the real situation and her daughter's real needs.

If her mother had been less hard core and approachable, my friend might not have ended up pregnant her senior year in high school. Everyone's worst fears were confirmed. It was a vicious cycle. I felt bad for everyone involved, but mostly I felt sad for my friend.

I had another friend whose mother was sick for a long time. Naturally, the whole family was upset and preoccupied. My friend was really shook up about her mother's illness, because she loved her so much, but she also had questions about sex—and she was thirteen. She didn't feel she could approach her father because she felt it was "indelicate" to ask about sex, things she really needed to know, when her mother was so gravely ill. She really did not want to ask him anyway. But, she couldn't possibly bother her mother with them, either, she felt.

My friend said to me, "You're so lucky. You can talk to your mother about sex." She needed to but she couldn't. I didn't have a totally calm adolescence and I wasn't always aware I was being "mothered" or "guided" or "educated," but I knew I was lucky not to be in the position my friend was.

Here's what I see as what a daughter may be up against when she wants to seek her mother's advice. I've also tried to suggest ways to get around the problems.

1. Her mother is deeply committed to a religion with strict rules governing behavior.

The area of religion is especially problematic. Many people rely on a particular faith and its accompanying values to guide them through life. When a daughter contradicts a mother's faith, this can understandably make the mother feel threatened, defensive and unreceptive to any kind of meaningful communication. The way to avoid this result lies in the approach to the discussion. A daughter could start a conversation about a facet of the religion that she questions by first bringing up the parts of the faith that she *believes* in. This at least puts the mother on a comfortable ground. Next, the daughter could begin to ease in to the religion's "taboo" subjects by asking questions about why the religion takes the position it does. The key is that the daughter must be aware that the mother is deeply committed to the religion, and that this commitment has strong roots. If a daughter really wants some answers, or at least a friendly discussion, she must keep in mind that religion and the beliefs it encourages are sensitive subjects.

2. Her mother has told her that sex or any kind of lovemaking is wrong, bad, sinful. She gets into a relationship and finds it's not so horrible, not that terrible. So she wonders if her mother was right in the first place and is afraid to go to her. Does it mean her mother lied?

In this situation, a daughter should try to understand that her mother hasn't lied, she has simply tried to protect her daughter from what she perceives as a threat to her daughter's well being. I don't think mothers actually label sex itself as a threat, rather, it is the *repercussions* that are so frightening: teenage pregnancy, social diseases, being outcast by peers, etc. Every daughter should think about the fact that if the mother really believed that sex itself was the evil, the daughter probably would not exist!

The daughter could attempt to alleviate her mother's fears by talking about how responsible she's trying to be about the relationship, how happy she is with it, and maybe even ask her mother's advice about contraception.

3. Her mother is embarrassed to talk about sex, as if it is something shameful. She hears the subtle and not-so-subtle messages and cannot bring up the subject.

I would recommend that a daughter start off by asking her mother about the first crush she ever had in grade school, or the first date she ever had and what it was like. What happened, was she nervous? The daughter could then turn the conversation around to her *own* crushes and questions.

4. She is starting to experiment sexually but her friends are not, so she may think she's doing something wrong. She doesn't want her mother to know.

Here, a daughter could describe what was beginning to happen, but at first say it was one of her friends going through the experience. One or both of the following should result:

The mother would figure out what was really going on and try to talk to the daughter about it in a supportive and informative way. Or, by talking about her "friend's" feelings, the daughter may become comfortable enough to reveal who the "friend" really is.

5. She's in a group at school that has always talked down about what other girls have done, she has done something like that, and thinks everyone will turn on her if they find out. So she doesn't mention it to her mother or anyone.

Again, the daughter could use the "friend" approach to try to open the subject for discussion.

The key to each situation is a willingness of both mother and daughter to be receptive.

The biggest barrier, I believe, is the question of parental credibility. The best analogy I can make is to compare parental warnings about the dangers of sex with parental warnings about the evils of drugs.

I am not a drug user, but I, too, have been told drugs are a horrible thing, dangerous, life-threatening and anti-social. Parents always warn kids about drugs. Despite the warnings, many kids are exposed to drugs early on, especially marijuana. They try them, and, usually, nothing happens, none of the threatened consequences occur: They are not immediately struck dead, nor do they instantly crave heroin.

So you have a kid who has been told all drugs are evil, don't do them. She tries marijuana anyway and ends up with relatively few bad results, nothing compared to the consequences she was told were inevitable. I believe drugs are damaging in the long run, but the reality is usually nothing compared to the warnings. The warnings are so out of proportion to what does happen that often kids go on and try something else, possibly more dangerous than marijuana.

They are in for trouble now, but there's also another trouble: They have lost confidence in their parents.

The same is true with sex. Many mothers want to protect their daughters from "going too far." Their warnings and threats become dramatic, but when their daughters find out these predictions were blown out of proportion, their mothers lose credibility and communication breaks down.

Mothers who are overanxious to protect their daughters from getting too involved, or, their worst fear, getting pregnant, warn their daughters that all aspects of love-making are bad, even kissing. And what happens is when a girl does kiss a boy, despite all the warnings, as girls and boys have been doing for milleniums—the girl thinks, "This isn't so bad at all. I don't find anything wrong with it."

Her distrust of her mother has begun. Like the little boy who cried, "Wolf!", prior warnings and future ones lose credibility. The result is a breakdown in communication between mother and daughter. The daughter understandably may hesitate to confront her mother by announcing, "You were wrong."

That's a shame. The daughter could have gotten good, helpful information from her mother, and the mother could have helped her daughter. Both mother and daughter lose.

I suppose I'm prejudiced because I can't understand why mothers wouldn't want to talk to their daughters honestly and openly, but I can understand why daughters wouldn't want to. It's hard for me to believe any mother wouldn't want input into her daughter's learning about sex, relationships and life.

Yet, I understand daughters who have a block against talking to their mothers about sex. Society tells them that sex is something to be ashamed of. Say you're a mother and you're ashamed or embarrassed about something you did. It would be hard for you to approach your daughter about it. You'd much prefer never to mention it. That gives you some idea why your daughter may be reluctant to approach you.

It's funny, I look and see a lot of my friends needing so badly to talk to their mothers about things happening in their lives, things they are really worried about, things that scare them. I look back and I don't see anything overwhelming, no shadows hanging over me. Maybe that's because I never let anything become too big a problem, that I talked about things as they happened, not only when I was desperate.

The best part is I always felt secure because my mom would be there for me when I needed her. I could always tell my mom.

IN THE BEGINNING

What are little boys made of, made of?
What are little boys made of?
"Snaps and snails, and puppy-dogs' tails;
And that's what little boys are made of."

What are little girls made of, made of?
What are little girls made of?
"Sugar and spice, and all that's nice;
And that's what little girls are made of."

MOTHER Contrary to that old and popular nursery rhyme, little girls are NOT made of sugar and spice, and little boys are NOT made of puppy-dog tails, either. These fanciful notions—which also lock little girls into being demurely passive and little boys loudly aggressive—were probably made up by Mother Goose because she just couldn't bring herself to tell her goslings the facts of life.

Telling kids what they are REALLY made of is much harder than that. And without knocking Mother Goose, who gave me and my children many happy—but carefully edited—hours of enjoyment, if you start out early avoiding the realities of life, it's going to be very hard to talk to your kids about their personal lives, their sexual relations when they get older.

If you are unable to tell your pre-schoolers that girls have vaginas and boys do not, and that boys have penises and girls do not, it does not bode well for critically important communication in the years ahead. When your children get to their teenage years or are old enough to be in college, you probably will not be able to warn them about the dangers of contracting sexually-transmitted diseases or the deadly Acquired Immune Deficiency Syndrome (AIDS).

Prevention is often the key to avoiding these health hazards. If you have trouble communicating on the entire subject of sex, you may not be able even to speak the necessary words of warning.

You simply won't be able to mouth the words. None of us *wants* to deal with this aspect of sexual relations, but ignoring it does not mean it will disappear.

Society's message today hasn't changed that much from the days of Mother Goose. Today, instead of sugar and puppy-dog tails, we talk about the double standard, which describes the same situation.

The dogma, without rhyme or reason, is that boys can do whatever they want sexually and girls cannot, that girls should be virginal until they "catch" a man and that "catching" a man is of the utmost importance. To do battle with this kind of propaganda, I felt I had to be very sure that I established in my daughter a strong sense of her own worth and control of her own destiny. I wanted to do the same with my sons, but I knew that society was on their side and it would not be a battle to achieve my goal.

My daughter, I knew, would have to be strong and confident to be able to decide for herself how she wanted to live and what she wanted to do, both personally and professionally. And, despite some of the negative aspects of society, she had some pluses going for her, too.

Cathy's gender was received with great joy by both sides of her family, a rather unusual reaction then and now for a first child. I was one of three girls and I therefore expected only to give birth to girl children. I was delighted with a healthy daughter and would have been ecstatic merely to have a healthy baby, but I felt a special pride in her gender because I *predicted* I would have a girl. My family was happy the all-girl trend was continuing.

Cathy's father had a brother and no sisters. The brother had three sons. So, on her father's side, the birth of the first granddaughter—it seemed she was the first granddaughter *ever* born to anyone in the world—was an occasion of great joy.

I don't think it hurt Cathy a bit that she always felt very important and very loved for what she was. The subtle, and sometimes not-so-subtle message that girls are less worthy than boys, was not given to her at home. Her complete acceptance and approval was a far cry from families who do not welcome girl children.

I think it's crippling to girls from infancy to know they are second choice out of two choices, and that they do not count because their families have the outdated notion that only male children can carry on the family name, business and ability to win sports trophies.

Most of my female friends, who were also busy having babies in those pre-amniocentesis days, told me they dreamed of having a boy as their first child. They also dreamed of their marriages lasting forever without any problems and living happily ever after. A male firstborn was an integral part of the fairy tale.

As crippling as this attitude is to the emotional growth and security of our daughters, it is still not so final as the treatment of some newborn female babies in India and China, where it is common practice to kill girl babies because they are viewed as a financial burden.

Gender and sex are two different nouns, and often confused, but in teaching my daughter about her biology I found them closely related. A child's attitude toward sex is shaped in the early years by those around her. A positive attitude is nourished by approval and acceptance. If she feels good about her gender, she will surely feel good about her body—at least that was the theory I operated on, by myself, in an isolated suburb in the Midwest.

Today, when my daughter tells me, "I grew up believing there is nothing I can't do," I feel very proud. And she has demonstrated that strength often. Her healthy attitude toward sex is an outgrowth of a healthy confidence in herself.

I have visible proof today that most of my instincts were right, but I wasn't right on everything. As most women in the '60s, I was groping my way to my own identity at the very same time I was figuring out how to be the best possible parent. The combination of the two shaped my approach to my children.

The surge of the second wave of the women's movement in the United States gave me great support. It also raised questions I had never considered. In retrospect, I didn't always make the right decisions—or I made the right decisions for the wrong reasons.

I believed then—and now—that self-image has a lot to do with everything that affects our lives, including sex. Yet, I named my daughter "Cathy." That's all. Just Cathy. A little girl's name. How could I expect her to be president of the United States with only a nickname for a first name? (This was, of course, before Jimmy Carter did it.) As soon as she went to college, Cathy rectified my error in judgment and named herself Catharine Elizabeth Kleiman, a strong statement of how she feels about herself: She wants to be taken seriously.

And while I'm confessing my sins—but only the minor ones—I decided to spell Cathy with a "C" and not a "K." Why? Because then her name would be Kathy Kleiman. And what if she married a man whose last name began with a "K", too? Then her initials would be KKK, and I certainly didn't want any association with that group.

It never occurred to me in those days, not so very long ago, that she might decide never to marry at all, and if she did choose to marry, might decide to retain her own name—or have her husband take hers.

Actually, the worst part of the whole name business was that I really wanted to name her Carol. I wanted to name her after me. But I couldn't do it. It seemed too egotistical. The fact that there is sometimes an extra psychological burden in life to have the same name as your mother or father was not my consideration at the time. I very easily named my first son Junior, after his father, and beamed with pride as I did it. I was once again deferring to the myth that the male of the family is far more important than the female, especially when it comes to "carrying on" family names. Naming my son after his father was a "natural" thing for me to do; naming my daughter after me seemed to be an act of self-indulgence.

Looking back today—with 20-20 hindsight, of course —I see the irony of my actions.

I also see how inappropriate they were. Today, I do not believe it's right to give children the same name as their parents, even though my reasons are completely different. I don't believe it's always psychologically healthy.

So my daughter's name is Cathy, and I did the right thing—for the wrong reasons.

When Cathy and her brothers were six years old and began asking questions about how babies are made, I started to talk to them specifically about sexual intercourse. I talked about it in what I hope was a relaxed manner, as if I had spent all my life explaining such matters. I never once mentioned the stork.

When talking to Cathy about sexual intercourse, I always used the expression "making love." That's how I felt about it myself, and I could not, no matter how hard I tried, use more sophisticated terms, such as "sexual intercourse," for instance. I was taking the easy way out with an euphemism, I suppose, but in retrospect I don't think I was all wrong: I transmitted my feeling that there should be an emotional relationship first, and that it is expressed to your partner by "making love." In my way, I made a distinction then between caring and not caring. The latter is what Erica Jong coldly described as the "zipless" form of sexual intercourse.

I faced head-on such words as "clitoris," "masturbation," "testicles" and "urethra"—words I had never heard, even once, in my house when I was a child. The proper words, believe me, were very difficult for me to utter as easily and with as much authority as "making love." But I forced myself to do it because I didn't want to trivialize the human body or sexual relations. The words became easier the more often I pronounced them, and, in that way, my daughter and I grew up together sexually.

My daughter—and my sons—were born in the '60s. If they had been born two decades later, I would have benefited greatly from reading the book, *Growing Up Free: Raising Your Child in the '80s*, by Letty Cottin Pogrebin. I and my friends were groping individually for the right answers. We did not know then that our isolation from each other—we did not discuss our deepest doubts with one another—was part of the problem.

Pogrebin's book could have bridged the gap for us in a way that Dr. Spock did not and could not begin to address, though I do remember telling everyone when my children were little, "Don't knock Spock!" In her book, Pogrebin, who has three children, lists what she believes is necessary for healthy attitudes toward sex.

The first is permission to feel sexual pleasure. Next, a positive attitude toward the body, your own and others. Also, the right to sexual knowledge without sex role distortions. And, finally, protection from sexual abuse, which Cathy and I discuss in the next chapter.

Women were just beginning to talk to one another honestly, at least a little bit, and, as always, sex was the most difficult subject. I remember one day when a friend of mine, a Phi Beta Kappa graduate of a distinguished university who also just had a baby girl, watched as I changed Cathy's diaper—certainly a busperson's holiday!

"You know," she said hesitantly, "I was really upset the other day. When I changed my daughter's diaper, she put her hands . . . down there." She pointed at Cathy's diaper.

"Oh," I said mildly. "What did you do?"

"I slapped her hands, of course!" she responded indignantly.

Her daughter was six months old.

I didn't lecture her on the lifelong psychological damage of forbidding children to explore and enjoy their own bodies, mostly because I didn't know too much about that. I did know that I felt my growing up not in touch with my sexuality was pragmatically an enormous loss of time, possibly a crime.

I knew my friend told me for reassurance, because she didn't feel right about her reaction. Our mothers, though, would have known what she did was the exactly right thing to do. But times were already changing. I told her my attitude was to give kids all the freedom they need, that all children masturbate because it feels good. I felt it really wasn't much of a problem.

"I never thought of it that way," she told me. "I was always told you went straight to hell if you masturbated. I'll have to think about it."

That's the best any mother can do: Think about it. Our personal beliefs and hangups are both our strengths and our weaknesses. It's impossible to ask us to get beyond them. We can only do what we can do.

The cultural lag—in what we have come to believe is acceptable intellectually and what we still have to understand emotionally—also handicaps us in our talks with our daughters.

For me, though I heartily approve of orgasms, to be able to discuss the subject with my daughter requires an act of faith that I'm doing the right thing. The hope is that it will be easier for her to talk about any and every aspect of sex with her daughter.

What kept me as honest as I could be is that I believe every word I said about sex in those early years had an enormous impact on my daughter.

That realization made me not only extremely cautious about my phraseology but also forced me, many times, to speak in the first place, though it might have been easier, in the short run, to remain silent.

DAUGHTER It would be nice to say that I remember every word my mother told me about the facts of life when I was very little. The truth is, I remember very few specific incidents, where we actually sat down and talked things over. What I do remember is the ease with which we discussed things.

One thing I don't remember, as I'm sure most adults—except for my mom, who never got an answer—would not, is asking about the differences between boys and girls or where babies came from. I am the only girl in my family and I have two brothers. Many of my friends when I was growing up were my brothers' friends. We were all close in age and we played together.

Often, I was the only female in a group of males. I knew I was different, but I was pretty-well accepted as a person, and I don't remember any specific hurts simply because I was a girl.

Occasionally, I felt left out when my brothers played football with their male friends—as my mother felt, too, when she was a child and her neighborhood friends left her out. But my feelings of rejection were *not* because I wanted to play football with them. They always tried to include me and I always refused because I didn't want to play.

What bothered my ten-year-old self was that my brothers wanted to do something I *didn't* want to do. I had the same reaction when they wanted to watch a different television show than I did. I simply wanted things my way. It was more a matter of stubbornness than anything else.

I do remember that sometimes my brothers went off and played and left me behind, but that didn't happen a lot. I was one of them. And when they did leave me out, I had my own group of friends, little girls, to play with.

What was good about this is that I always felt comfortable with and accepted by both girls and boys. This has carried over to the present time, because I have several close friends who are female and several close friends who are male.

I was always aware that I was a girl and I liked being one. I preferred it. Perhaps part of it was that I felt singled out as being the only daughter. I liked the attention. But I also liked being the same gender as my mother, which my brothers, of course, were not. If anything, I always felt special.

Today, the experts would probably call that sex-role stereotyping. I always identified with my mother, and I was only aware that some of the things I did with my girlfriends were different from what I did with my brothers and their friends.

No one ever made fun of me for being a girl, so I always had a sense of personal worth. I knew I was an equal and was never taught to defer to boys. I can't remember a time I didn't know the two sexes were different biologically, but the boys accepted me—and I accepted them.

This kind of closeness, as I remember, underwent a few changes when I was in the fourth or fifth grade. It had something to do with physical differences and with the fact that my girlfriends and I were beginning to spend much more time together. It was suddenly "not cool" to talk to a boy or be seen with one or hang around one. All boys in the Lyon Elementary School had "cooties," as far as the fourth grade girls were concerned.

I think that was the time the girls got together in their

groups and talked about where babies came from. I have a feeling the boys did the same. We were now more openly aware of our biological differences.

I certainly never felt that my body structure was inferior to a boy's, but I do remember when we'd all be out playing, if my brothers had to go to the bathroom it was real easy for them. All they had to do was go off and go to the bathroom in the bushes—but I couldn't do that.

That's one of the few differences, not just in physiology, but in practice, that I was aware of.

I remember the talks we had in school about sex, the exhibits we saw on the development of a fetus, the television shows on childbirth and the books my mother read to us about sex. I also remember when she reviewed a Swedish book on children's sexuality for her newspaper. It was called *Show Me!* and created quite a stir. My mother interviewed me and my brothers about it, and wrote about our reactions as we read the book and looked at the graphic pictures of naked children playing with themselves and each other.

I was very young at the time, probably only ten, and some of the photographs surprised me. But my comment for Mom's story about how her children reacted to the book was not that kids were not ready to read it, but that "probably, *parents* are not ready for a book like this."

I also said that I didn't learn anything from it I didn't already know, which was probably not quite true. And, I added, for publication, that I didn't "see what all the fuss was about."

Today, I suspect that the book probably wasn't written

for young children but to titillate adults—pedophiles—who got their kicks out of seeing children naked. With what I know today from reading so much about child pornography and child abuse, I think it was probably a pornographic book.

However, my reactions to the book show I wasn't the least bit upset by it, was confident enough to take it in stride and didn't giggle and laugh when I read it, as some of my friends did. I remember being matter-of-fact about it.

And something else, too: I wasn't the least bit embarrassed to read it with my mother and brothers. My friends were shocked when the article appeared in the *Chicago Tribune*.

"How could you look at that awful book with your mother and your brothers?" one of my friends asked me in horror.

"Why shouldn't I?" I replied.

In retrospect, this incident shows me that at age ten, the basic groundwork my mother had tried to lay was already in place: The mention or portrayal of sex did not frighten me. It was a fact of life.

As sophisticated as I seemed to my friends, it actually took me a long time to understand where babies really come from, even though I was certainly told often enough.

Knowledge of sex came to me little by little as I was growing up. Learning about sex, I believe, cannot be taken out of context. Sex was never held up to me as some big, red banner that could ruin my life or make or break a relationship. It was never highlighted to me as being extremely negative, either, or something to avoid.

I can imagine it would have never worked if my mother had tried to do a story on my friends' reaction to *Show Me!*.

I don't think they could have expressed their honest reactions. They might have said whatever they thought that she, as an adult, would want to hear. They probably would have been able only to express their embarrassment —but not their interest.

I have no doubt it would have been a good story, the one the editors were expecting, if one of us had said, "This book is absolutely disgusting. It should be banned."

It's purely an individual thing what little girls want to know about sex, how much they remember of the answers and how aware they are of the physical differences between girls and boys.

Mothers, no matter how well-meaning they are, can't force their daughters to talk to them about sex if the daughter isn't ready, especially if she's unsure about how she feels and is not ready to admit her uncertainty.

I guess it's up to mothers to try to gauge how willing their daughters are to talk and to what extent. Not an easy task, but worth the effort.

Now there are very good books on the specifics of sex. If you have a video cassette recorder, there are some excellent videos on the subject, too. There's nothing wrong with buying them for your daughter.

Offer to read the books with your daughter, if she wants you to. Offer to watch the video with her. If she doesn't want you to, let her watch it alone. Either way, some kind of intimate conversation is sure to follow.

A concept as large and encompassing as how life begins takes a while to absorb and to accept. I'm an adult now, but there are several things about sex and sexuality I'm still sorting out.

My mother gave me a strong base from which I can ask questions, of myself and others, mull over the answers and come to my own conclusions. That's what little girls *should* expect to get from their mothers. Most of society, even today, two decades into the so-called sexual revolution, does not heartily endorse the way I was brought up. Many mothers still believe that moral judgments and rigid rules are what they should, as responsible adults, teach their children. It is ironic that I am the most conservative person among my peers when it comes to relationships and sex— and *I* never heard moral judgments or rigid rules.

Fortunately for me, my mother gave me many gifts. One of them was a direct approach to sex. And since she started this chapter with a poem, I want to end it with one, Dorothy Parker's verse, "Godmother."

In the poem, Parker talks, in the way only she can do, about the christening of an innocent baby.

The good and saintly godmothers give the new baby girl all the virtuous traits they believe she will need in life, the traditional truths. But another godmother, a hag, the "bad" one, shows up at the hallowed event and gives the baby "sadness and the gift of pain, the new-moon madness and the love of rain."

After the "bad" godmother's gifts, Parker observes, it did *"little good to lave me / in their holy silver bowl, / after what she gave me / —rest her soul!"*

STRANGER DANGER

MOTHER | Today, mothers are aware of the dangers of child abuse and kidnapping. We cannot rid our minds of the images evoked from the television show that told the story of five-year-old Adam Walsh, whose severed head was found floating in a canal in Florida. Additional warnings from advertisements on television, public transportation and milk cartons remind us about the dangers our daughters, like Adam, are vulnerable to from strangers.

More quietly, the message is being publicly spoken that strangers aren't the only threat to our daughters' well-being. People they know very well—fathers, brothers, uncles, family friends—can also do harm. These terrible truths present mothers with a very tricky assignment:

We have to give our daughters enough information about sexual abuse to keep them safe—yet not make them fear all men.

I worried that I might go too far with my heartfelt admonishments and terrify my daughter so much she'd be afraid to go anywhere alone. I was also concerned that the many accurate and justified warnings she might hear both at home and in elementary school would send another message to her: To fear, mistrust or hate all men. A delicate balance was necessary to preserve her emotional growth and protect her from potential physical danger.

In the '60s, when my daughter was born, no one gave little girls specific warnings. "Stranger Danger" was taught occasionally in some school settings. My children's grade school was one that did, but the talk had only a single message to impart: Don't get in anyone's car if you don't know the person. Some teachers also warned not to take candy from strangers. Their concern was to prevent kidnapping; nothing about sex was mentioned or implied.

Child abuse, incest, rape and battered women were subjects not spoken out loud in those days—at least not in public and certainly not in front of the children.

Yet the statistics we know today, such as the fact that one out of three girls younger than eighteen have reported incidents of sexual abuse, certainly prevailed when Cathy was growing up. I, for one, do not believe the numbers are necessarily increasing today. What is increasing is women and girls are finally talking about what happened to them. And that's the best thing that can happen as far as our safety is concerned: Problems kept secret don't get solved.

Cases of sexual molestation are severely underreported. Kids don't always tell their parents and parents don't always tell the police. What's of extreme urgency to most mothers, and it certainly was to me, is to make sure our daughters know what might happen and how to protect themselves.

The first moment I held Cathy in my arms, I admit I did not think of ways to warn her about sexual abuse.

But one feeling I had was so strong I can still feel today how it coursed through my body then: "Nothing must happen to this precious child. She *must* be safe."

There was nothing unique about my emotion. It's called maternal love. How to implement that protection without keeping my daughter within eyesight every moment and without causing her nightmares was the problem. Some of my friends, also deeply concerned about their daughters, settled for dire warnings, no matter what the effect might be on their little girls.

"I don't care if she *is* terrified," said one of my friends, after telling her daughter that Big, Bad Men lurked on every corner. "I just want to keep her alive."

There seemed to be a great deal of commonsense in that philosophy. Adam Walsh's parents would have settled for that.

Closer to home, we had our own horror story: We knew of a family whose five-year-old daughter had been kidnapped and raped on the way home from kindergarten. After weeks in the hospital having her torn insides repaired, the little girl returned to her home and school. She was lucky. She lived. But neither she nor anyone else in her family was ever the same. I imagine they are still haunted.

"Something" happening—that was the fear in my heart. I thought long and carefully how to communicate realistic warnings to my daughter without imparting the paralytic dread I felt.

Lucky for both of us, I realized early on that dire warnings alone were not sufficient protection. I had to give Cathy confidence in herself and pride in her body; those two characteristics are strong weapons in handling all forms of sexual abuse, from being offered rides by strangers to molestation and incest.

Because of the urgency I felt for Cathy to see herself as a complete and worthy human being, I quickly developed an antagonism to fairy tales. It seems to me that the most popular ones tell girl children to be submissive and dependent and that they are victims who can only be saved by men.

As we learn more and more about the extent of child abuse in our society, it would seem to me that it would have been just as sensible, in many cases, for Red Riding Hood, Cinderella, Snow White and Sleeping Beauty to have been saved *from* men.

Susan Brownmiller in *Against Our Will* describes the tale of Red Riding Hood as "a parable of rape." Jack Zipes in his important book of contemporary feminist fairy tales, *Don't Bet on the Prince*, gives this synopsis of the oft-told story of the little girl, her grandmother and the wolf: "A little girl is raped and is made responsible for the atrocious act."

Whereas I had carefully edited the nursery rhymes to include girls as well as boys, I had to revamp drastically the fairy tales I read to Cathy. In the story of Red Riding Hood, I tried to downplay the little girl's desperation and vulnerability. In my house, Red Riding Hood runs to tell her mother about meeting the Wolf. Her mother immediately calls the police, some of whom are female, and they arrest the Wolf. Then she, her mother and grandmother all go out for pizza.

Cathy used to laugh at my version of the stories; she knew I was doctoring them, but not why.

Tired of struggling with the so-called "happy" endings of passivity and obedience, I quickly switched to *Where the Wild Things Are*, in which Max was just as often Maxine when I read it. I read Cathy *Winnie the Pooh* and *Charlotte's Web* and books by Ezra Jack Keats and Louisa May Alcott— books I liked to read myself.

Cathy's safety, I believed, lay in her not expecting a Prince to come along and save her. She was an adored child but not raised to be a fairy Princess. I tried to teach her to be herself. From the time she was a little girl, Cathy was aware of my "propaganda" and often dismissed what I had to say. When she got older, she often fought back, saying, "Mother, you're weird!" Still, she heard.

In this way, her self-confidence grew. It encompassed many things, including dealing with the idea of sexual abuse. I had problems here, too, that I often felt inadequate about: I wanted her to recognize sexual abuse and to cope intelligently with the frightening prospect of it. But I also wanted her to understand that if something did happen, it was *not* her fault.

It's not Red Riding Hood's fault that the Wolf attacked her. We should not blame the victim for the crime.

Girls and women who are raped did not "ask" for it, were not in the "wrong" place and were not dressed "inappropriately." The person at fault in all these instances is the rapist, the attacker. So once again, I was on my usual parental tightrope, trying to balance teaching Cathy to be aware of danger and also making sure she understood bad things can happen to good people who are completely blameless.

I used to change songs and lullabyes, too. I'd sing them the "right" way first and then add my variations. In "Rock-a-Bye, Baby," I'd let the cradle and baby fall first. Then I'd sing:

When the bough breaks,
The cradle will fall,
And Mother catches baby,
Cradle and all.

Mary had a little lamb and so did Robbie and Rayme. "Blue," *she* was a good dog, too, now and then. The farmer in the dell was often female and took a husband, despite dropping corn prices. These were my efforts to adjust the balance of power, to empower my daughter as my sons were.

I was far more successful instilling a sense of self by reading to Cathy than singing. I don't have a singing voice. Even as toddlers my children would ask me, "Please, *don't* sing!"

Because it had never been done for me, I was sensitized to the importance of not gluing feelings of guilt and shame to sex. Many mothers tell their daughters how terrible anything connected with sex is and then are very hurt when something untoward does happen and Mother is the last to know. What did they expect?

Many girls would rather conceal sexual abuse than risk what they suspect will be the wrath of their parents, too.

I feel very fortunate that when a man exposed himself to Cathy and her friends in the school yard, Cathy remained calm and came home and told me about it. She'll tell you herself about the incident, later in this chapter.

I was so proud of her maturity, even though she was only nine or ten years old. I immediately called the police. I, a non-violent person who does not believe in capital punishment, would gladly have done this man serious harm. I didn't show Cathy my fear, but I showed her my anger. When we talked it over, I told her she had done what was best for herself and that she should feel good because perhaps this would stop him from doing the same thing to other little girls.

Even though she did not fully understand how dangerous the situation was, Cathy knew how to handle it. What would I have done as a child? I would have been the perfect victim because I knew little about sex and nothing about it as a form of aggression.

I still remember something that happened to me when I was in the second grade. A classmate asked me to play "Doctor" with him. We went to his house, into his bedroom and closed the door. He then explained the game: He would be the doctor and examine me. Then I would be the doctor and examine him.

I agreed to play. He said he would be the doctor first. I undressed and he examined me thoroughly, with his eyes only, never touching me.

"Now it's my turn," I announced.

"No," he said. "I don't want to play anymore. Go home."

I went home crying. I never told my mother. Sexually, nothing much had happened, but I was upset because I had been tricked. I felt powerless, ripped off, taken advantage of. I learned little about sex from the incident. In retrospect, I tell myself the moral of the story is: Go first. The real lesson, which no adult explained to me, was not to let anyone take advantage of me sexually. Cathy knew that in elementary school.

Many years later, I heard that my former classmate had become a gynecologist! I roared with laughter when I heard it and wondered if he was giving me any credit. And then I began to worry about *why* he became a gynecologist.

If your daughter knows her body is hers, to be respected, she will not let people take advantage of her. She will not be intimidated. My daughter and I talked about the little girl we knew who had been raped. Not every detail, but that it was a crime and how sad we were about it. Since we talked about so many things, my warnings weren't out of context and didn't frighten Cathy; instead, she became informed.

As I mentioned earlier, I feared Cathy would distrust men or think I did, especially after her father and I were divorced. But all by herself, my daughter has learned to judge people, including men, individually.

Knowledge is power, and power is protection.

Cathy now has a finely-honed sense of what's right and wrong for her. She quickly detects insincerity. She senses when other people are playing games and she abhors it. She has such a strong moral guide, molded for her own person, that I always say, "I want to be just like her when I grow up."

Cathy is indeed grown up now, and sometimes when I don't quite approve of her decision to do something, or do not totally adore one of her buddies—all I have to do is look askance, and she'll look me right in the eye and laugh and say, "Trust me, Mom."

And I do.

DAUGHTER | Looking back and remembering the days when I was in elementary school, I can see how difficult it is to warn little kids about the dangers of sexual abuse and not scare them to death at the same time. Ever since I can remember, my mother always explained to me what could happen and what I should do, but despite all this information and awareness, I was incredibly naive.

I knew a lot and I also knew very little. I also firmly believed that nothing bad could ever happen to *me*, even though I knew things that had happened to other little girls. I think the best example of how most things having to do with sex are so highly-charged with emotion is a somewhat minor incident I was involved in the third grade.

It happened in the school yard, after school. Ironically, my mother was always so pleased that the lot she chose for our house to be built on was adjacent to the school yard. The back of our house faces a modern elementary school with 3½ acres of green grass, ball fields, basketball courts and playground equipment.

My mother, who worked as a reporter full time from home for many years, could watch us go to and from school from the kitchen window because the school path is also adjacent to our house. Mom could even see us when we played in the school yard—quite a contrast to the way she grew up. Mother lived in a tiny row house with no back yard, only an alley, and had to walk over a mile each way to school, crossing busy streets. She always told us how glad she was that we didn't have to do that, especially in cold weather. All she had to do was push us out the back door and we were in school—and she knew she didn't have to worry about our ever getting hit by a car on the way.

But a school yard also attracts a lot of creeps, especially after school. My mother cautioned all three of us to keep away from strangers—to *run* away if necessary.

I remember being warned both in school and at home about things as basic as not to take candy from a stranger and not to trust people you don't know just because they're offering you something. Usually, they want something in return.

That's a good general rule to remember, for mothers to tell daughters.

No one told me exactly what to do should a man expose himself, but I really believe that no one, including my mother, expected anything like that to happen in our pleasant suburban neighborhood. I certainly didn't. We all felt safe.

The warnings put me on guard, but I don't think they dented me or did any serious psychological damage. There really is a fine line between saying "don't trust anybody at all," and saying "just be careful."

And one day I did put the warnings to use.

I was playing in the school yard after school with three of my girlfriends. A man came near us and exposed himself. I didn't know it was exposure but I knew enough to get out of there as fast as possible.

My three friends became hysterical, crying and screaming. The man ran away. I ran home to my mother —it was a short distance and I got there very quickly. I told her, "Mother, there was a man in the school yard going to the bathroom! It scared my friends."

That's what I mean about being naive: I thought he was going to the bathroom and that's what I reported. I was not upset as my friends were because I didn't perceive any danger to me. I thought it was something not so harmful as it really was. I wasn't frightened at all, which may or may not have been a good thing.

The flashing lights went off in my head warning, "Go home. Tell your mother." So I did.

I have to admit I didn't even feel uncomfortable about what the man did because I knew what to do: Disappear.

My concern was for my friends and their reaction, which, in retrospect, perhaps was more appropriate than mine.

My mother looked very upset when I told her and she called the police. So did the mothers of the other girls. Within a few moments, the man was picked up and arrested in the school yard. My three friends had to go to the police station and pick the suspect out of a line up.

I never got called in by the police and I was so glad I wasn't. I didn't want to deal with it—although I did, in my own way. After that, the school yard was patrolled regularly by the police. My mother told me the man was either masturbating or exposing himself in public, which are against the law. She said he liked to intimidate little girls and could be dangerous.

Everybody still talks about how I "handled" that situation with such maturity. I think I was *lucky*, the way things turned out. Maybe I had too much trust. Maybe I was too "comfortable" about the whole thing. Whatever it was, the basic communication both my mother and I have stressed so much was in place and worked: I told her. If I told her for the "wrong" reasons—because I underestimated the situation —that probably wasn't too good for me. But I'm glad I never had to find out.

Though I did tell my mother about that incident, I didn't tell her *everything* that happened in my life. I kept plenty of secrets from her not only about sex but all aspects of my life. You just can't tell your mother everything. I knew of things that happened to my friends and I never told my mother about them. That would fall in the category of betraying a confidence, and as long as I felt I could deal with stories I heard of someone "touching" someone or other things like that, I felt no need to discuss them.

When things bothered me, such as our friend's rape, I asked my mother a lot of questions. And I got answers.

I have to point out that my mother was eternally vigilant, not in a domineering way, but always listening to what I said and sometimes hearing more than what was there.

I remember one vacation when we drove to Florida. On the way, we stopped in Nashville, Tennessee, and stayed at a motel with a swimming pool. I was about eleven, my brothers, ten and eight. There was a lifeguard and we were good swimmers, so mother let us swim without her. Still, she was nearby, and I ran to tell her something wonderful.

"Mom, mom, there's a boy with 'peenies' in the pool!" I told her, imitating his Tennessee accent and his word for 'pennies.' I was excited because he threw pennies in the pool and my brothers and I were allowed to keep what we dove for. "Look at what he gave us," I said triumphantly, showing her a handful of coins.

Mother was on her feet and at the pool. She thought I was saying, "penis," and was ready to do battle to protect us against the miscreant who was giving us pennies to do who knew what. We still tease her today about those "peenies."

With all I knew, heard and read, I still did some of the things I was warned against. Sometimes, I and my girl-friends would hitchhike, even though I knew, in my mother's eyes, at least, that meant instant death.

I was about fourteen then and my friends and I thought it was cool to hitchhike now and then. "Everyone" did it. I never told my mother about it because I knew she'd have a fit.

My friends and I got away with it, the few times we hitchhiked. I guess we were lucky. I always knew it was wrong and that added the element of danger to the excitement of doing such a daring thing. One day—of course, I never hitched at night; I wasn't that dumb—a neighbor drove by and stopped for us. She drove us home pleasantly enough and never gave us a lecture or even indicated there was something strange about two young girls standing on the road hitching a ride.

But I knew my number was up, and I was right.

My mother was furious when she heard about it. "You could be killed, raped, kidnapped! Is that what you want? Why don't you take the school bus that I've been paying all that money for?" She really carried on and broke all the rules she had tried to establish for equal communication, without lecturing, threatening or moralizing, between mothers and daughters.

I already knew what I had been doing was stupid, but she yelled at me so much I wasn't ready to admit it, or to promise to stop. "*Everybody* does it," I said. I knew that was one of the excuses that drove her wild.

"Well, *you* are not going to be one of them," she yelled. "*You* will be different. *You* will get to live, even if I have to stay home from work to put you on the bus myself and make sure you take it home."

Then, to my surprise, she began to cry.

"Cathy," she said. "Please don't do anything to harm

yourself, anything so foolish as hitchhiking. I couldn't bear it if anything ever happened to you."

"Okay, Mom," I said reluctantly. "I won't hitchhike anymore."

"You'll be sixteen in a couple of years and you'll be able to drive then, just make sure you get to live that long."

"All right," I said, as she calmed down.

Having won that battle, she quickly began her next campaign. "And remember, when you are the driver, don't pick up any hitchhikers. They could look as innocent as you do, but still be dangerous."

I promised. And when I was sixteen, sure enough, my mom bought me a car to drive myself and my brothers back and forth to school. It was a small, inexpensive car, that I used to joke was probably made of paper.

It also occurred to me that driving in that subcompact car was probably more dangerous than hitchhiking, but I was so grateful for such a munificent gift, I never pointed this out to my mother. A lot of people thought I was much too young to own my own car—even if it saved three expensive bus fares and my mother's sanity.

A lot of her friends told her when she got me the car she had done the wrong thing. For the right reasons.

What mothers have to realize from the anecdote is that no matter how much you warn your daughters, they are still going to do what they want to do, not to upset you or to endanger their lives, but just to make their own decisions.

That doesn't mean there's anything wrong with the warnings or the information. There isn't. You just have to be ready to hear it. Some girls will rebel against the idea of always having to watch out, having to circumscribe their lives because of dangers they are prey to merely because of their gender.

Even if that's not the message intended, it's still delivered. It's true, too, but that doesn't make it easier to accept. Because it includes not only school yards and cars, but going out alone at night, to the movies or a restaurant or anywhere.

Some of the warnings push young girls in the opposite direction from where mothers want them to go. They purposely defy all orders from "above." Others, are so frightened they verge on being agoraphobic. Though some parents prefer the latter because there are so many true stories of kidnapping and child abduction, neither is a healthy reaction.

I know some parents who prefer their daughters to be "too" scared. I know others who prefer their daughters to know nothing; they hope innocence will be bliss, even though it rarely is.

And though I was warned about some men, I never related the warnings to fear of *all* men.

I was told never to talk to strange men; I was never told not to talk to any man.

I was well informed, but I have no fear of men. I don't have close relationships with people unless I know them very well. We have to be good friends first, with time for a certain level of trust to build, before I really open up.

I remember being warned about strangers and realizing there could be a danger to me from someone I didn't know, but it hasn't negatively affected my later relation-ships with people, including men.

Stranger Danger was just another facet of my world, a world I'm comfortable living in.

THE BIRDS AND THE BEES

MOTHER | Speaking of sex to a pre-adolescent girl is not the easiest assignment for a mother brought up in pre-sexual revolution days. And I am one of those mothers.

How simple everything would be if we could just sit down with our young daughters for one day—we could make it a major holiday and call it "National Birds and Bees Day"—and tell them everything we know and want them to know about sexual intercourse, orgasms and the meeting of ovum and sperm. Those who find details of sex too embarrassing to articulate face-to-face could sit behind a curtain. NB&B Day would be obligatory, a Constitutional requirement, a condition of being a good and patriotic citizen—maybe even tax-deductible!

What's most attractive about this idea is that it would have federal sanction and the whole thing would be over in twenty-four hours. But we all know it's not that easy. A one-shot, marathon session won't do it. It takes, at the least, sixteen years of close communication.

We're handicapped in many ways in telling our daughters not just where babies come from, but how they got there in the first place. Sex is one of the few things we teach our children without showing them how to do it.

I've demonstrated for my daughter—and my sons— how to make a bed with a hospital corner, my own approach to loading the dishwasher, how to dry each lettuce leaf for the perfect salad and how to watch sports on the television screen while listening to the play-by-play on radio. I've shown them, by my own example, that you do not cry when you've lost an important tennis match until you get to the car, that you never lend money—you *give* it to the person—and that it is important to be active in causes you believe in.

All these matters are far less complicated than sex, yet no one would think of explaining them without doing it. Actually, I was far more familiar with the shapes and contours of lettuce leaves than of my own body. I still remember how shocked I was when a friend of mine called from Los Angeles where she was attending a Women's Self-Help Health Clinic. "We used mirrors and examined ourselves!" she announced with glee. "I never looked before. I expected to find stalagmites and stalactites growing!"

Cathy was about twelve at the time and I told her the

story as an amusing anecdote. I explained women don't know what their vaginas look like because we've never examined them. I told her our ignorance was due to shame and warnings of never to touch, but that the human body is beautiful, including the vagina—despite jokes to the contrary.

I did not follow up by saying, why don't we take a look together, as some mothers might. That was beyond me. I didn't ask my daughter if she had ever examined herself: Her sense of privacy was already too strongly established for that.

In the '70s, women were beginning to get married later, to experiment sexually, to understand their own sexual desires. Women and men were living together in greater numbers—and admitting it. I feel that today's statistic of twenty-six million heterosexual couples living together is greatly undercounted: I believe it represents only the couples who will tell their mothers. There are probably many more.

Today, the marriage rate in the United States is at its lowest level in a decade. Baby boomers are marrying later and less frequently. But that doesn't mean they're not having sexual relations and that makes sex education, at an early age, essential.

When I was growing up, there was tremendous pressure to remain a virgin until marriage, when all the mysteries of life would be miraculously revealed by a loving husband. His sexual "condition" was never articulated, but the assumption was that he would be an experienced lover who would make the heavens open up and, at least, the earth move.

Nothing was ever said forthrightly, and certainly even the word "virgin" was not mentioned. But the message was strong: Ignorance was the only path to bliss and security. My mother tried to keep me safe, in the only terms she knew. This lack of acknowledgment of sex, female sexuality and sexual experimentation outside the institution of marriage went out the bedroom windows in the '70s as the sexual revolution peaked—even before television shows such as "Dallas," "Dynasty" and "Falcon Crest" and R-rated movies brought a new aspect to the concept of Show and Tell.

Messages about sex, many of which I disapproved, bombarded our home through sexually-explicit magazines, books, television shows and movies that degraded women. I wanted to make sure that Cathy not only learned about sex, but that she knew the difference between healthy sexuality and pornography and other putdowns of women.

In my "birds and bees" lectures, I gave my own version of right and wrong. I told Cathy never to do anything so obscene as to enter a Miss America contest or to pose nude for a centerfold. I told my daughter and sons that *Playboy* and magazines like it are destructive of women—even when the contorted photos are sandwiched between "quality" articles. Playboy degrades women by making us sexual objects. The marketing of flesh, which is usually female flesh, causes male contempt and violence against women, I told them. Like war, obscenity and exploitation are not healthy for children and other living things.

I corrected them if they used words such as "slut," or "cheap" when referring to women. I explained these words reflect a double standard. I still remember my mother cautioning me when I was twelve years old that only "cheap" women wore their hair in bangs. Of course, when she said that, I immediately snipped off my long pigtails, which I still had, and cut my hair into bangs. In my own way, I was trying to make my own decisions—to do what I wanted to do.

I tried to lay the groundwork for my daughter to be nonjudgmental of sexual activities that do not harm others. She is far more conservative than I in many of her attitudes toward sex, but is strongly in favor of individual rights.

Even though my lectures frequently covered the technicalities of penis being inserted into vagina, or vagina receiving the penis, of sperm fertilizing egg or egg absorbing sperm—the basics of sex—I never knew if Cathy really understood what I was saying. But it was clear she heard.

I explained these details without too much embarrassment because I was so certain of their importance. But I never mentioned another important ingredient, passion. Passion is the vital energy of sex, a driving, exciting, encompassing emotion that deletes concepts of time and space. No bed should be without it. I couldn't mention passion or lust or desire or craving or wanting. For some reason, the subject of desire embarrassed me. And I have suffered the consequences of not expressing myself honestly in this matter: Now that my children are young adults and I so much want to tell them about the pleasure and insanity of passion—it's too late. They won't listen. And when I insist upon speaking my mind anyway—can you imagine trying to explain what President Carter meant when he said he had "lust" in his heart if you have not previously mentioned the word?—my children listen with tolerant amusement, but do not hear.

I did mention orgasms, but not too often because they were another thing it seemed to me that Cathy didn't want to discuss. I did announce that there is no such thing as a mutual orgasm and that vaginal orgasms are the invention of men, not the reality of most women. I did mention that women often faked orgasms to please men and that there can be a certain emotional pleasure in doing so—but it is certainly not a sexual one. On occasion, I would say that women should stop faking and start enjoying orgasms, that we are entitled to them, the same as men.

I wanted my daughter to know she didn't have to be a passive recipient, as I had been until recent years. I sometimes would say to her: "A baby is living proof that only one person has to have an orgasm to conceive." My comment fell into the category she labeled as "weird." But she understood what I was saying.

The joys of oral sex, especially for women, was an area I could not talk much about. I didn't know how to and she didn't especially want to hear it from me. But she knew I liked it. She also knew I thought babies were wonderful when you wanted to have them and that childbirth is hard labor.

We didn't discuss masturbation openly, either, but she knew I thought there was nothing wrong with it and never associated it with shame or disgust. Once in a while, I might comment that masturbation does not make warts grow on your hands, but that was the extent of a verbal message. My silent communication was making sure each of my children had a bedroom of their own, a place to be private and alone with themselves.

In the early years, sex was easier to talk about because I was a married woman, with the status and societal approval that title implied. But when Cathy was seven years old, her father left and we were subsequently divorced. The impact of divorce was harder on me than on her—I hope. It hurt me to talk about lovemaking, commitment, romance, all of which I had mentioned frequently and enthusiastically in the past.

Now I was a single woman, dating because I felt I should be, reliving some of the anxieties of my teens and 20s—this time with the additional responsibility of three children under seven. After a decade of marriage, in which I took sex for granted, there was none, unless I went out looking for it. I felt betrayed as a woman and betrayed as a mother. I now was fully in charge of the raising of my family, the only parent apparent.

I was angry, as well I should have been. Yet, I wasn't angry at all men and I wasn't bitter. I wasn't opposed to the idea of love or the act of sex. They just seemed rather remote at this point in my life. Still, I talked to Cathy about love and marriage, even though I determined to stay away from both for as long as possible. In fact, I have stayed away from marriage, but, fortunately, not from love.

Within a year or two of my divorce, most of the original shock and pain had passed and I began to date more frequently. I never became too seriously involved with any-one because I was basically still numb, still committed to my non-existent marriage. I don't know how much the children understood of what was going on. I think they saw my grief, whether they understood it or not, but they felt secure in the fact that I adored them and would never leave them. How could I, without a babysitter?

Despite the fact that I believe Sigmund Freud is as dangerous to women and girls as the nuclear bomb is to all people, I watched my children, especially Cathy, who was the oldest and female, for any signs of psychological dam-age. I never found any negative ones, but still I looked and was especially vulnerable to criticism in this area.

Though I start each day by saying, "It's not my fault!", I think, in those early days of divorce, I had a twisted notion of letting my children down, somehow, by not providing a full-time father for them. I know now, and can prove it, that what is needed is at least one caring parent of any gender. That one caring parent, as it not so surprisingly turns out, is usually the mother.

When Cathy was eleven and her brothers ten and nine, something happened that made me realize I really didn't have to worry, that their psyches were strong, and that I—as a divorced woman—had not embittered their attitudes toward life. It was a wonderful, albeit hilarious, discovery.

One evening, my friend Sherry called to tell me she and Dick were getting married. I had introduced her and Dick and both were grateful to me for doing so. I was among the first to know of their marriage plans and they wanted to share their joy with my children, too.

I put each child on the phone to hear the happy news. Ray and Rob were unimpressed with the announcement, but Cathy was clearly perplexed.

"Oh, no," she told the happy couple. "How could you do that?"

Her reaction upset them, especially Sherry, who explained they had fallen in love and then asked Cathy to put me on the phone. "You must be doing something wrong for her to react that way," my friend told me. "Whatever it is, you've got to stop or your daughter will be harmed all her life."

She questioned me as to whether I was badmouthing men or making fun of marriage. Did my children ever see me in a loving relationship with a man? I claimed I was innocent of trying to twist my daughter's mind against men, but still . . .

Sherry had the solution to the problem. "We're going to have a small wedding," she said. Sherry was widowed and Dick divorced. Both had teenage children. "But you will have to come and bring them with you, so they can see what love and romance is all about."

The wedding was planned for August, during the time I and the children were going to a Michigan resort for a week. "It's not that far away, you can drive in for the wedding," Sherry insisted.

Though I never really doubted myself and never felt guilty, I thought I'd better do as she advised, just in case. I wanted to make sure my kids got the message that the wedding was a very important occasion. I bought Ray and Rob their first suits, neckties and new shoes. I bought Cathy a lovely long dress, black patent leather Mary Janes and frilly socks. I bought myself a lovely summer dress, too.

The day of the wedding was bright and filled with sunshine. It was hard to drag the kids away from the lake and to get them all dressed up, but they understood this was a very important day to me and cooperated without too many protests. We got in the car and drove back to the wedding at Sherry's apartment.

The children and I were seated on the front row. Everyone fussed over Cathy, Ray and Rob. Everyone spoke to them of love and marriage. Sherry and Dick had written their own ceremony, someone played guitar music and the couple's teenage children were involved in the ceremony. There was a lot of love and a lot of food. My children looked very impressed and happy.

We drove back to Michigan and on the way I kept saying how beautiful the wedding was and isn't love wonderful. Cathy and her brothers were in the backseat and were unusually quiet. I continued with my programmed litany of how romantic the day had been. In fact, it was.

Finally, Cathy leaned forward, poked me in the back and said, "Mom, about the wedding. How could they do it? Isn't is awful?"

My heart sank. I thought, Oh, my goodness, I did this all for nothing. I've ruined these wonderful children for life.

"What are you talking about, Cathy?" I asked her.

"Didn't you like the wedding?"

"I liked the wedding," she said thoughtfully, "but how could they do it? They're too old. They have gray hair!"

I laughed so hard I almost drove off the road. It was simply a case of prejudice against age, not against love between the sexes, not a reaction to an embittered parent.

That experience taught me an important lesson. As I explained to Cathy and her brothers that gray hair doesn't necessarily mean you are old, or too old to love and marry, or too old to enjoy sex, I resolved never to feel guilty again.

About anything.

DAUGHTER | During my adolescence, which my mother claims went on for nearly a decade, I tried to put two and two together to figure out what people did one on one.

Even though sex was never a hidden topic in my house, I often wondered why it was a secret in my friends' homes. They talked a lot about what their parents "did," and if their parents really "did it." Most of my friends knew what it takes to make a baby. They just couldn't believe that their Mom and Dad actually performed such an embarrassing act.

I had been told the facts a million times. I was told them about women and men. The birds and the bees were not mentioned. Still, I only listened to as much as I wanted to, and I only heard what I could comprehend at the time. My mother made a supreme effort to educate me and my brothers about sexual relationships, but nonetheless I had many staggering misconceptions, as most kids do.

My mom is horrified when I tell her I was convinced for a long time that babies were delivered to your doorstep, not unlike the mail.

Then, also for many years, I thought the only time you could get pregnant was during your period. I believed that that was why women had their periods—so they could know exactly when they were fertile and able to make a baby. It seemed incredibly convenient. I have no idea where this misinformation came from. All I know is I truly believed it, as did my friends. I have recently learned that it is one of the most common misconceptions young girls have.

I don't remember my mother being pregnant—I was less than four years old when both my brothers were born—but I do remember seeing pregnant women and being aware that they were carrying a child. I observed their penguin-like figures and I heard their complaints. I also heard their joy and anticipation, but I wondered how they could stand being so uncomfortable and if I would ever be able to. I thought about it a lot because I look forward to having a family of my own.

My mother never minimized the discomforts of being pregnant or the real hardships of childbirth, but she also told me that both were wonderful, exhilarating experiences. Because she was truthful about the negative parts, I believed her about the positive ones; her approach is one I hope to imitate some day. Today, I have a balanced view on pregnancy: It's undeniably difficult, but worth it.

Despite the openness, at least verbally, in my house, I definitely wondered what my parents did in their bedroom with the door closed. I didn't think about it excessively, though. I just accepted it as part of the bigger picture. I accepted the secrecy, too—sex was something my parents did in secret, away from me and my brothers—as not so much hidden or mysterious, but properly private.

My mother bought me a lot of books on sex and I don't remember one of them. I do remember a television show we all watched on the birth of babies. I remember it was graphic and explicit. I was grossed out by it. I wasn't ready. It was just like the films they showed us in elementary school. I always looked away during the part where the woman was giving birth. I was too young to appreciate it as a natural part of life.

I had no desire to watch these films and so I didn't. Today, I realize I was turned off by the mechanics of delivery, of blood, sweat and toil. They showed the woman pregnant but never really explained how she got that way. I suppose they were doing the best they could to teach us about sex within the framework of the school and the times, but the films skipped the parts of pregnancy that I was curious about, and I blocked them out.

My fourth grade girlfriends and I often speculated on the possibilities of how a woman *became* pregnant in the first place. The films always started with an egg and a sperm: We wanted to know what the woman and man were *doing*.

I always enjoyed reading Judy Blume's novels and her

recent nonfiction, *Letters to Judy*, is as on-target as her fiction: The letters from kids today ring true for me and the time I was growing up.

Blume notes in her book that kids don't want to know about their parents' sexuality. They want the heavy stuff kept private. All kids want is reassurance that they are normal, like everyone else. And Blume makes this statement: If you can talk with your kids about sex, you can talk to them about anything. But are they listening?

To this day, I have no specific memories of being sat down and told where babies come from. It was an ongoing exposure and learning experience.

It is the nature of adolescence that mothers and daughters grow apart at the same time they physically grow closer. There are many misunderstandings at this time, some minor, some major. My mom and I had plenty of them.

Some of the minor ones were the "peenies" in the pool and Sherry and Dick's wedding. While working on this book, we've found a few more. Mom told me how impressed she was that when I was only ten years old I bought her *Our Bodies, Ourselves*, by the Boston Women's Health Book Collective.

"Cathy," she told me, "I couldn't get over that you had found that book before I did. Actually, I should have bought it for you, instead of your buying it for me. Where did you hear about it? You were so precocious!"

"Thanks, Mom," I replied. "But I had no idea what the book was about. I merely asked a friend of yours what to get you for your birthday and she suggested *Our Bodies*. So I bought it for you."

At the age of fourteen, I was fairly rebellious. I wanted to be my own person. We have a family photo that is symbolic of me at the time: My mom, brothers and I are standing on the steps of the Field Museum. Mom and my brothers are standing very close to one another, smiling. I am off from them, a little bit to the right, and I am not smiling. I look angry. I was.

I was deeply moved by *Coming of Age in Samoa*, by Margaret Mead. That was a book I read in a high school anthropology class and gave to my mother to read. I told her, "If we only lived in a different culture, we'd understand each other so much better." My mom read the book and agreed with me.

Today, she quotes to me from a book by Sheila Kitzinger, *Woman's Experience of Sex*. The author says that the "need to assert a separate identity may happen partially because there is nothing in our society that allows the formal and cumulative acquisition of status as a girl moves into womanhood, as in the past, when she let down her skirts and put up her hair . . ."

The rites and the passage of time today are far less distinct and therefore more explosive. Truthfulness between mother and daughter is basic, but it's not always enough. My mother has not lied to me. She's never suggested sex was only meant to produce babies; she taught me to respect my body, not just for sex or as a potential incubator but because it was mine to live in and enjoy; she never perpetuated the myth that woman have to pretend they are virgins until they get married. Still, I often felt alienated from her. Today, I know it's a part of growing up, becoming my own person.

All teenagers go through turbulent times. Compared to my mother's adolescence, mine was placid: She practically tore her house apart. Still, more than a few of my mother's friends tactfully suggested that perhaps I was "acting out" because I came from a "broken" home.

Nothing makes my mother more angry than that word. Just because a father wasn't present doesn't mean we don't have a close-knit, loving family. My mom made it that way, and so did my brothers and I. Our house was always a home, despite divorce, and that's why my mom is my number-one role model. She really showed me that a woman could do it all, and she showed me at a time when it was unusual for a woman, much less a single parent in the suburbs in the Midwest, to succeed the way she did.

I was disgustingly normal. My parents' divorce was a stressful, traumatic thing, but it was the only major upset in my childhood. I look back to those times and I search for catastrophic events, but I can't seem to find any. All I can think about is that everything was just so normal.

When I was very little and Mom told me she and Dad were getting a divorce, I said, "Oh, no, isn't it enough we're the only ones on the block against the Vietnam War and President Nixon?" I was very upset about my parents' splitting up and that my father would not live with us anymore, but I also didn't want to be different. "We're the only people I know who are divorced," I said to my mother accusingly.

We may have been the first, but not the last, and

within a few years I had many friends who lived in single parent homes. Still, divorce was pretty much a novelty, and some of my friends whose parents weren't divorced felt sorry for me and for my mom, too. When Mom began to date and show up at various school affairs and parties with men, my friends and their families were very curious. Mom told me she was often the topic of a lot of gossip, but that she didn't care and I shouldn't either. She thought it was funny.

I was never queried about my mother's sex life, which I suppose was what the speculation was all about. People asked me, "Well, is your mother involved with anybody yet?" They wanted my mom to have somebody, a man to depend on, like they did. They wanted her to be happy, in their terms.

Everyone always asked me if Mom was "seeing" anyone. I didn't feel they were prying. They were just worried about her being alone at a time when women were not alone.

I suppose if I had really been precocious at that time, as my mother sincerely believed I was, I would have thought, "My mother has some nerve going out and dating, just when I'm beginning to be so interested in men. She's a grown-up. She has no right to cut into my adolescence, to go through some of the same things I am."

Some of my friends—both boys and girls—felt that way about their divorced parents, but I never did. I was always glad when my mom was interested in a man because that meant she had someone to divert her from her concern about the divorce. I was always glad when she seemed to like a man.

Sometimes, we'd go on trips with mother and a male friend and I never thought of it as a problem. It was wholly acceptable to me, or at least I never questioned it. My mom was happy and that is all I noticed. My brothers and I liked the extra attention we got. Mother always told us—and still tells us—she doesn't plan to remarry, so we never felt threatened.

My mother and I have discovered another misconception. About this time, I had the feeling my mother always wanted to "Find Somebody." She'd always point out to us in restaurants or at school events, "Oh, look, isn't that a nice family? There's the father. Isn't that nice?"

I remember those comments, and the message I got was that my mother was somewhat envious. Today, she explains to me that she wanted us to know that fathers can be responsible for their families, too, loyal and attentive. I interpreted it as a longing on her part, so I was always relieved when she was involved with somebody nice.

I don't think my attitudes toward sex were affected negatively by my parents' divorce. I was affected, but in what I consider a positive way: I am very wary about relationships and am very careful about whom I get involved with. This has stood me in good stead.

Another effect of the divorce was that my mother was always so busy I sometimes had the feeling I could get away with a few things other kids might not dare to do in a two-parent household. Something weird happened that proved me wrong—and also showed how close my mom and I are.

One summer when I was fourteen—the big year for my rebellion—my mother told me she had a date to go to a cocktail party Saturday night in a suburb about an hour from our house. Then she was going out for dinner. Immediately, I decided to have a party. I didn't tell her a word about it, but I began inviting a few friends from junior high school.

Saturday came and Mother and her friend left for the party. In the beginning, my friend and I had a good time and everything was under control. But as it began to get dark, the word spread, as it does when there's a party, and before I knew it, total strangers were coming to the door. Some were older guys—old enough to drive. They came in vans and pickups. At one point, I didn't know 75 percent of the people at my own party.

The older guys brought plenty of alcohol and that's when I began to panic. The party quickly became unmanageable. I wanted to leave but I knew I couldn't. My brothers were frightened as people began to spread through the house, though I had told them they had to stay downstairs or outside. Boys and girls went into the bedrooms. The party was completely out of control. I knew what was happening wasn't right and I wanted out. But I was helpless.

At the very moment I was about to become hysterical, my mother and her friend walked in the front door. I was scared and very relieved. Mom got everyone out from the downstairs part of the house; her friend went upstairs and systematically cleared the bedrooms. As the kids came downstairs, Mother stopped them and got their names.

Within fifteen minutes, the nightmare was over. But what was Mother doing home? How did she know? She explained she was at the cocktail party and felt uncomfortable, but she didn't know why. She said she and her friend went to dinner, ordered their food, and when it came, she simply stood up and said, "I'm sorry. I can't eat. I have to go home. Something's wrong." They paid for the uneaten food and left.

Can you explain that? I can't. Neither can she. I was certainly calling for her in my heart, but how did she know? She says we're tuned in to one another, and other things have happened since that indicate we are. Thank goodness! Mother treated the party as a home invasion, not an orgy, but she did call the parents of every child in the house and in the bedrooms, both girls and boys. She told me that one of the mothers had called her own daughter, thirteen, a slut.

I'm an adult now and give parties when I'm home in the summer without telling my mother, but they are under control and she doesn't mind. Well, not too much! I learned a lesson from that experience and she knows it: My parties are carefully planned and supervised. If something would go wrong, though, my mother would probably receive my anxiety signals. Call it intuition, extra sensory perception, astral communication—whatever it is, my mother has it when it comes to her kids. And she watched us as closely as two parents.

I hate to think how that party might have ended. I was ashamed about what happened for a long time. And rightly so. My mother emphasized the importance of my being responsible, personally and as a member of the family. But she also told me not to wallow in guilt forever.

"Remember," she comforted me, "there are one billion people in China who don't know about your party and don't care."

I recall those words even today.

WHAT OTHER MOTHERS AND DAUGHTERS SAY ABOUT SEX

We talked to scores of mothers and daughters about what they tell each other about sex and what they don't. They present a United Nations of American women—rich, poor, middle class, and from all geographic areas of the United States.

They range in age from eleven to fifty years. They are Black, Asian, Hispanic and Caucasian and come from multiple ethnic backgrounds. The women are from all economic classes, too. Their sexual orientation includes heterosexuals, bisexuals and homosexuals.

We didn't do a scientific study with strict statistical boundaries. We're not scientists. We just talked and talked until we got a crosssection—perhaps a patchwork quilt is more accurate—of how mothers and daughters feel about sex, love, marriage, babies, birth control, abortion, homosexuality, divorce. And just how much of that they share with each other.

We found that once the mothers and daughters agreed to speak with us, they spoke frankly and honestly. Many of their stories are deeply moving: Sex is the cornerstone of many of the emotions of growing up, and also of many of the painful facts of life.

Mary told us up front she was relieved her daughters didn't tell her much about sex. Frances said she thinks premarital sex is a sin. Sallie had an abortion and never told her mother, though she still wants to. Eleanor learned when she was ten that her father wasn't dead—her mother had never married.

Gretchen had been married, had children and was divorced when she realized she was a lesbian. "And I never even had a crush on my high school gym teacher!" she says. Margaret, who also is divorced and has a live-in male lover, feels sorry for women who are not bisexual.

Nancy, who describes herself as having been "promiscuous"—forty-five lovers in one year—says when she was young, her mother flaunted her sexuality in a damaging way. Charlotte didn't get an abortion because it was illegal; today her daughter is the joy of her life. Peggy says her mother doesn't always tell her the truth about her own sex life; her mother, Maureen, is proud of how open she is with Peggy.

These are some of the feelings mothers and daughters have. You'll read them in this revealing chapter. We have included six sets of mothers and daughters together.

After that you'll find four additional interviews with mothers alone. We did not interview their daughters because they did not want their daughters to know some of their most intimate—and potentially hurtful—experiences and feelings. And some of these mothers didn't want *their* mothers to know all about their sex lives, either.

We've also included interviews with four daughters— unrelated to the four mothers. They, too, wanted to speak openly and could not if their mothers knew their identities: They didn't want to hurt them or strain their relationship.

We've changed names and other identifying facts to protect the women kind enough to cooperate, to share their innermost feelings in the hopes of helping other mothers and daughters to communicate better about sex.

One thing we did not change or mask: Each woman's deep love and concern, her awareness of the difficulty of talking about sex and its enormous power in her life and in her relationship with her mother or daughter.

We are grateful for their many voices, which enrich all of us and help us to keep afloat, add to our buoyancy in the turbulent waters of mothers and daughters speaking of sex.

We are deeply moved by their self-searching and desire to relate exactly what happened—their very own facts of life. Unbelievable as it might be, the stories of their lives are true. They told us of joy and excitement about sex; they also talked about being battered, abused, about fear.

The stories we've chosen to repeat here are facts of life only mothers and daughters know.

Mary is forty-eight years old, has been married twenty-five years and has four daughters. Martha, the second oldest, is twenty-one.

MARY | I never told my daughters the facts of life. Maybe I was a little bit afraid to. I thought that if they had questions, they would ask me, and they did. In fact, I only remember discussing the facts of life with Martha, when she went off to college. I don't even remember what I said.

But I know what I believe and I definitely feel that there should be no sex before marriage, that you should not get that seriously involved. Sex is a rather sacred act. At least, when I was growing up it was sacred. I was taught it's against the Bible to have sexual relations if you're not married, and my kids do know I feel that way.

My oldest daughter, who is twenty-four and married, lived with her husband before they were married. I told her, I can't say I like it, but *please* don't get pregnant till you get married, and she didn't.

I wasn't told anything about sex or periods when I was growing up. My daughter Martha learned from her friends. She told me she had started and I made sure she had the right equipment, but she didn't even ask me why she had a period, what it was all about. Obviously, she already knew.

We downplayed sex in our home, but my daughters know I would like them to have what I have, a great bunch of kids and a fine husband. I've been very lucky in my marriage and never do I take anything for granted. I don't know what's going to happen tomorrow.

I've never discussed abortion, either, with my daughters, but I feel that it's up to the person involved. I don't know how they can make laws saying a woman can't have an abortion if she wants one, especially if it's a rape case or she physically can't carry the baby.

That being said, I know abortion is something I would find very hard to do myself, but that's hardly a problem anymore. I am truly happy I was married during the wild years of hippies and all the sexual freedom.

I do hope my three single daughters find nice men and get married. I want them to be married. I think they have high standards because of their father.

I know my kids are strong and secure. We worked hard to bring them up that way and with a deep religious and moral faith. I don't worry that they might do something wrong sexually, something they'll be sorry for all their lives. That's not a worry. But I do have a tremendous fear of their being hurt.

I don't want my daughters to be hurt.

MARTHA | My mother never sat me down and told me about the facts of life, but in the fifth or sixth grade in school we had a big thing on sex education. She told me about my period after it had happened. I learned a lot from my friends and from my older sister. My sister told me any time I had questions I needed to ask and I was too embarrassed to go to Mom, to go to her. So I did.

But I learned a lot from my family without being told in words. We're a big family, very loving, and I know how my parents feel about things. I am very close with my mother, but I don't tell her everything. I tell her some things. She usually remembers them and sometimes fires them back at me! I like it when she does that.

I'm not dating right now. I just graduated college and I'm back home now. I do see one friend occasionally, but it's nothing serious. I can't date casually. I can't go out with more than one guy: I can't keep them straight. Since college, I haven't met anyone I'm willing to become involved with.

Sex is not that important to me. It's important in a relationship, but it's not the main thing. In my high school class, sex was no big deal. We were never that sexually interested. We went to football games; we had fun.

You get yourself in a position to be hurt if you're not prepared for a sexual relationship. I don't think a lot about birth control but I do have a couple of friends who were put on the pill to regulate their periods. It's hard to know what's safe.

Abortion is a really hard issue, but I believe it should be a woman's choice. Nobody else should make that decision. If you've been raped or the baby has serious defects and you know for sure, it would be okay then. It's not good to have a baby born who is unwanted and abused. But I don't think you just go out and have fun and then get an abortion to get it over with, to get rid of it. Abortion is a tough topic but it's for women to decide. I don't think the Big Heads [male legislators and judges] should make the decision for you.

Even though we don't have specific talks about sex, I am very close to my mother. My mom depends on me and I depend on her. I can tell when Mom's upset and she knows all about me and what I feel. If I didn't tell her something very personal and important that's going on in my life for more than a day, I'd burst!

I want to be like my mom. She's a homebody and I like to travel, but when I have kids I want to settle down, like she has done. My mom is the greatest lady who ever lived. I'm so lucky. All my friends come home and want to adopt her. She's so open and willing to hear new ideas and is always there for me.

I think daughters should be honest with their mothers, not hide things and not lie. I'm very private, even with my mother, but I would let her know if I were involved with someone, if it were serious.

And even if I didn't tell her, she'd ask! She wants to know—and then she hedges a bit because she respects my privacy.

Gretchen is fifty years old and is divorced. She is a lesbian. Her daughter, Beth, is twenty-six.

GRETCHEN | When I was an adolescent, my father was intrusive. I can't say I was physically abused or a victim of what is traditionally known as incest. But he did violate my privacy by constantly interrogating me about sex. He had a prurient interest in my sexual activities. And that violated my privacy and my sense of worth.

I was heterosexual and was married for eight rotten years during the '50s. I was heterosexual until I was divorced and moved to a new city, where the men available were really creepy. My male lover was in another city and was involved with other women. That hurt me.

I joined several women's groups and met some women who were lesbians. After a year, in which I got to know some of them, I realized that what was available were first-rate women and bottom-of-the-barrel men. I couldn't deal with men politically anymore, it was always a hassle. And some men were violent with me.

I began to be interested in women. It didn't seem like an outrageous thing. I absolutely had no interest in women previously. Growing up, I had no crushes on any girls. I never even had a crush on my gym teacher! Only on boys.

My first relationship was wonderful. It was long term.

After the first time we made love, the first time I had a homosexual experience, I thought, "How nice, I never have to perform fellatio again!"

I didn't tell my daughter. I didn't discuss it with her. But she knew. Other people told her. She never asked me. Then, my lover and I talked about living together, in my home, sharing a room, a bed. Before making that decision, I went to a psychiatrist and asked if it would harm my daughter. I was assured that if this was something I wanted to do and was comfortable with, there was nothing to worry about. When I said I was sure my daughter knew but didn't ask questions, I was told not to shove it down her throat, that if she didn't want to see it, she didn't have to.

I did tell my mother, who lives in another city, because I was going to be in that area for awhile. She said she already knew, that she had figured it out by herself.

Even though I, my first lover and my daughter lived in the same house for several years, Beth didn't ask questions. When she was little, I talked to her about sex and told her the facts of life. I even showed her my diaphragm and spoke to her about contraceptives.

When my daughter was a young teenager, I knew she had boyfriends. She didn't tell me she was having sex, but I assumed she was. I always encouraged her to bring her boyfriends home and I let her go in her room and shut the door. I didn't want her mugged in the park.

I think my daughter was more embarrassed by my political ideas than my being a lesbian. She didn't like the posters and slogans I had in the house, especially in the living room.

Even when she was older, she didn't want her friends to come over and see my weird posters. She didn't want her wedding reception at our house for that reason.

I don't think my being a lesbian has hurt my daughter or confused her sexual identity. It actually uncomplicated my life. When I came out, my life was simpler. I admit I did have good male lovers, but I was tired of breaking them in. I always felt as if I was teaching Sex 101.

It was good for me to get involved with women because I like women better than I like men. Men are in a group that oppresses women. I've never slept with a Republican of any gender. I have to approve of the politics of the people I sleep with.

I found it easy to have sex with a woman and I would tell my daughter that, if she asked. I was orgasmic with men but always had to worry about at what point to have an orgasm, about keeping a delicate balance.

There's a lot of fear—and it's realistic—about sexually transmitted diseases. Lesbians are the safest people in connection with AIDS. The safest person to have sex with is a lesbian who is not an intravenous drug user.

I hope my daughter fulfills as much of her sexual potential as possible within the constraints of society. I would be happy if she were a lesbian. I'm happy she's happily married. Women with sons are lucky in a way: When they get married, they get a daughter.

I love my daughter. She lives far away from me and I miss her. Despite the distance and the fact that we still don't discuss our sex lives, we are very close. Mothers and daughters have very special relationships.

BETH | My mother did not tell me about her being a lesbian. I suspected something. I probably felt too self-conscious to ask. She must have felt uneasy, too, because she didn't say anything to me. She wasn't open about it and I think if she had been real open and obvious about it, I might have freaked out a little.

I never thought that I might become a lesbian because my mother was, but when I met my husband in college, I didn't tell him for the longest time. I guess I was afraid he might think less of my mother. We were talking about Mother in some other context and I guess I must have finally said, "She's gay, she's a lesbian." And he said, "I figured that out."

I have a clear recollection of when I was in elementary school and my mother talked to me about the mechanics of sex, how babies are made and menstruation. I got the message from my mother that my sexuality was in my hands, and as long as I didn't feel used and didn't get pregnant, what I did was my decision.

When I did become pretty heavily involved with a guy, I told her. I talked to her about birth control and she advised using foam and a condom. I was only sixteen and really very prudish. It was awkward for me to go into a drugstore and buy foam. So my mother went in and got it for me. I love her for that.

About the same time, I read *Our Bodies, Ourselves* and found out all I could about lesbians. I wanted more information. The book said that everybody is basically both homo- and heterosexual, that our feelings go both ways and it's not terribly unusual. I relaxed a little then.

I was pretty sure I was attracted to men, but when I

went to college it was hard for me to initiate any contact. I was too scared, and they disappeared. I was bouncing off the one serious relationship I had in high school, which broke up, but not on my initiative. I needed another companion to fill that gap, and fortunately, I met my husband.

My mother was very responsible, I think, in caring for me. She made my first appointment for a gynecological checkup and kept making them for me until I got married. I have a three-year-old daughter, and when I was pregnant I asked Mother a lot of questions, which she answered.

I did want to get married. Very much. And I wanted to have children. I want for my daughter many of the things my mother wanted for me, primarily that she not be used in a relationship. Actually, today I feel pretty conservative about sex. Sometimes I think I have a double standard. I would not want my daughter to be involved sexually as early as I was. You really have to be emotionally mature. It's a heavy thing to handle.

That my mother is a lesbian is not the determining factor in our relationship. She is so unconventional anyway that I have been affected more by that: I want a traditional marriage and to be a standard mother. I got much more flack for the stands she took than for her sexual orientation. It wasn't so much her being a lesbian as those whacky pictures on the wall.

Dorothy is forty-five years old and has
been married twenty-three years. She has three
children. Barbara (Bobbie), her only daughter,
is twenty-two years old.

DOROTHY | I wasn't very curious about sex until I was twelve years old and got my period. My mother gave me a little book called, *Growing Up and Liking It*. I had functional questions about my body, how it worked, what menstruation meant, but I didn't have a lot of concern about having sex. It was never even an issue because my mother made it very clear that I was expected not to have sex until I was married.

Things like orgasms, birth control and abortion were never mentioned. We were so strongly indoctrinated not to have sex before marriage that it made it a lot easier, growing up then—much easier than it is for kids today—because there were no options.

The emphasis was on being popular and going out on a lot of dates and I was lucky because I was popular. I was very proud that no one put a hand on me; I wasn't that kind of girl. I wasn't involved sexually with anyone when I was a young teenager, but I wasn't a virgin when I got married.

I was nineteen and still living at home when I had my first sexual relations. I didn't tell my mother because there was no point to it. She wouldn't approve. I felt very comfortable; sex was a natural part of a relationship that was intense. I didn't worry about birth control. The boy used condoms—I didn't know how smart I was then!

I'm not sorry my mother didn't tell me every detail about sex. I wasn't ready for it when I was fifteen. She did teach me how vulnerable you are when you're emotionally involved, and that was more important to know.

Still, I wanted to be much more open with my daughter than my mother was with me. I think Bobbie knows that. I discussed sex with her all along, but particularly as she was getting ready to leave for college. I urged her to be friends with a boy first and then try to get a handle on how that relationship would change if they had sex, how she would feel if they had sex and he didn't call her the next day. It's very different from a goodnight kiss. Figuring that out hasn't changed from when I was growing up. I'm realistic enough to know most young women her age have sex, I just don't want her to be devastated.

Since she's been nine years old, I've answered all of Bobbie's questions about sex to the extent she was ready to hear. I answered generically, because I think sex is very private and there are certain things daughters and mothers do not talk about comfortably. Yet, she talked to me freely about the things she heard in school. We talked in an open and natural way.

I asked her a lot of questions. She's living out of town in a studio apartment and mentions male friends. I ask if the men stay over. Bobbie says, how can you ask me that? I reply: I'm your mother. I can ask anything.

There is nothing she can do sexually I would disapprove of in terms of morality. I just don't want her involved in anything that would drain her and leave her hurt. She is highly competent and extremely intelligent. She handles her life with sensitivity and good judgment. I have every confidence that extends to sexual behavior, too.

I feel terrific that my daughter can talk to me and I can talk to her, with no taboos. But we are two autonomous people and have strong feelings and thoughts about privacy. Her father and I have every confidence in her.

BARBARA | I remember my mother telling me about the facts of life. I was about eight years old, maybe a little younger, I don't remember precisely, but I do remember vividly that we were on vacation and I was in the bathtub and Mother was sitting there, watching me, waiting for me to finish. I asked where babies come from. Maybe it came up because we saw a pregnant woman, I don't know. But I do know she answered all my questions.

By the time I got my period at age fourteen, I was thoroughly prepared. We sent away for some booklets when I was ten and I read them about sixty times. I thought they were wonderful. But they didn't explain sexual relations, just plumbing. There were photos of female reproductive organs and how menstruation occurred. I remember being worried because all my friends had their periods and I didn't. My Mom assured me I was normal and that things like that are hereditary to some degree. That made me feel better. And she was right.

Today, we talk about everything, but as far as explicit sexual experiences, we are both fairly private. I don't know what she shares with her close friends but with me she is private and I'm private with her. But all along, when I've had burning questions, she has answered them.

I wondered what my mother and father did. They grew up in a time with generally understood taboos about sex. I wondered if they adhered to them, or broke them and lied about it.

It's crucial, particularly for the only daughter or an only child, to be close with your mother. Friendships aside, the primary relationship is still with your mother. It's more than learning about mechanics and specific feelings associated with sexuality. The best thing you get out of a mother-daughter relationship is the openness, the ability to communicate and the sense of self-esteem a good relationship with your mother can give you. That really helps you in sexual relationships and in your friendships.

I've learned from my mother that sex is a very important part of life. Right now, I'm making earth-shattering career decisions and that's taking a lot of my energy. Relationships, just at the moment, are not the main focus of my life. I have felt differently in the past but only when I felt in control, in charge of my life. I'm no good to anyone else when I'm not feeling independent.

The way I feel now, I'm a much better friend, so I'm not involved. Whatever I do, I know my mother understands.

Maureen is thirty-six years old and recently divorced.
Peggy, fifteen, is the oldest of three children.

MAUREEN | I feel I'm very open with my kids, especially Peggy. She was very receptive to talking about sex until she entered puberty, which is rather typical. You can talk to kids about a lot of things as long as it has nothing to do with them personally, doesn't threaten them.

I had my tubes tied before I was divorced. I didn't tell Peggy then, though she knows now. She was too young. I was sterilized because my marriage was breaking up. One night I dreamed I was pregnant and woke up in a cold sweat. I thought, what would I do if I got pregnant? I never ever wanted more children under any circumstances, I could not think about dealing with an abortion and I was so poor then. After my divorce, I knew I'd be even poorer.

I was divorced just as Peggy was entering adolescence, so I tried to be very straight with her about sex. I remember my mother telling me about the facts of life when I was nine. It was clinical: She told me I was going to get my period. She never mentioned orgasms or anything like that, but I was so uncomfortable and embarrassed.

I remember someone telling me the way you have babies is you did it with your doctor, which made sense. I was kind of surprised when my mother said you did it with your husband.

When I was divorced, I didn't date at first. Today, my sex life is limited, but whatever I have, I don't have it at my home. I don't know it would harm my children, but I'm a little uncomfortable with the concept. Besides, I like to make noise.

I don't worry about me. I do worry about Peggy. Last year, she told me she was involved in a relationship. I wasn't shocked, I was worried about her. She had been close with the boy for a long time and was very depressed when it broke up. I wanted her first experience to be wonderful, but I guess that was unrealistic. I've tried to talk to her about birth control but she doesn't want to talk to me about it.

I'd like Peggy to be autonomous long before I was: I want her to have good sex, mutual enjoyment and not to settle for putting out in exchange for love, support or money. Trusting somebody makes for better sex. It's the dimension that makes it more than masturbation.

PEGGY | Whatever I've asked my mother about sex, she's always told me. I started asking in the first grade. She didn't tell me all the details. I found out stuff later, when I was ten. I always looked at books.

When I got my period, she was the first person I called. She was at the office and was real excited. I was real excited, too, because I was first among my friends. I had to be the first. I was always the leader of everybody. I wanted to be older, to get a bra, to French [kiss] someone. But I'm scared now. I still wish I was twelve. When you're older, you don't have any fun. I don't know what's going to happen.

Mother never really gave me any rules about dating at first, when I was eleven or twelve. I didn't know anything. Then, last year, I started getting rules. She told me I was not allowed to see someone I had been involved with for a long time. I was obsessed with him. He hurt me, a lot. She didn't want me to be hurt. So I sneaked out to see him. I don't tell her about him anymore. I keep it to myself.

If I ever get involved with someone again, I won't tell my mother. Sometimes I'll tell her if I kiss someone, but more personal things are private.

I haven't had enough experience to know what's the best kind of birth control to use, but I would use it. If my mother knows I'm seeing a guy, she'll come to me and mention that I should think about using birth control, going on the pill. I wouldn't want her to know if I'm having sex with someone. It's embarrassing. I might tell my friends, but not her, though if I had a real problem, I'd go to my mom.

I think everyone has the right to abortion, but I don't think it should be used as a form of birth control. My mother believes in having the baby and giving it up for adoption, but she would be supportive of whatever I might decide to do. She told me last year she had her tubes tied. It bothers me because she hides a lot of what she does from me, and then she tells me how open she is with me, that she has no secrets, that we can talk about anything.

Mom tells me she's just good friends with a lot of people when it's really more than that. She tells me you should be in love before you have sex, but she goes to bed with people she's not in love with. I'm happy she has a sex life and isn't walking around frustrated. She's a normal person. But it makes me mad: She tells me one thing and does the opposite.

Elizabeth is twenty-nine years old and has been married eleven years. Her daughter, Jennifer, is ten years old.

ELIZABETH | I learned about the facts of life in a strange way and it's influenced my life and that of my daughter's. My older sister got pregnant when I was seven years old. My mother said, "Don't ever do that. Don't let a boy come near you. That's what happens."

So my first sexual information was negative and powerful. It made me very boy wary during adolescence, and particularly wary of a particular type of male, one who was poor, lower class and from a black neighborhood.

Even though I am black, this sounds racist. But what my mother was trying to talk to me about was the perpetuation of the underclass. She told me if you got pregnant, you ended up on welfare, that it's a trap you get into because you have nothing better to do. We were very poor and I didn't have many choices. I opted for education, to stay in school, to pull myself out.

So I turned off my hormones and turned on my brains.

I was a virgin until I was seventeen years old. It was someone I knew and loved and had been dating for two years. I was in control of the relationship. I wish all women's first sexual experience—and especially my daughter's —would be as wonderful as mine. He was a man who cared as much about me as I did about him. He tried to make it beautiful for me.

Surprisingly, it didn't seem all it was cracked up to be. I didn't know what orgasm was but when I found out, I still didn't have any. It was an age of sexual freedom and a proliferation of sexual information. Every woman can but I couldn't. I found that while I had no guilt about having sexual relations before marriage, I did feel as if there were something wrong with me because I didn't have orgasms.

I didn't become orgasmic until after I was married at nineteen—and not right away, either. Then I went hog wild!

With Jennifer, I have always been casual, open and honest. I've taught her that sex is a natural and loving act that means responsibility as well as pleasure. When she was almost ten, she got her period, and we celebrated it. We toasted her into womanhood.

She understands, in a far more positive way than I did, that menstruation is tied into being fertile. There's not much at ten years that girls today don't know. At age ten, she thinks the notion of sex sounds yuckie. It's not associated in her with urgings.

When the urgings do come, I hope she'll talk to me about birth control. I will not be judgmental or moralistic. I just don't want her to be a parent too soon, and I suppose I have that in common with my mother.

We've talked about masturbation, too. I became fascinated with myself at age ten, looking, touching. I spent hours doing that. My mom said that while it wasn't wrong to masturbate, it shouldn't be done in public and that I might get an infection!

Jennifer went through a period of secrecy in which she jumped under the covers when I went in her room. I told her there is nothing wrong with masturbation. In fact, I told her, it is medically wise and physically healthy to be acquainted with your own body.

She still wants her privacy, though. She throws me out of the bathroom. She says, "You may have diapered me when I was a baby, but I didn't have pubic hairs then."

We talk about things I never talked to my mother about.

Jennifer and I have talked about abortions, homosexuality, sexually transmitted diseases. About abortion, I tell her I believe every woman should have the right to have an abortion for whatever reason she chooses, even if it's an irresponsible one. It should be legal and affordable. My daughter disagrees. She looks at it this way: What if you had aborted me?

What isn't true for her that was true for me while growing up is a major fear of pregnancy. What I hope for her is that she gets involved in sexual relationships that are mutually caring and sharing. With me, sex always had a stigma, because of my mother's warnings not to get pregnant. My daughter knows that I approve of being pregnant when you want to be and can embark upon it with the right human being.

Today, you can get AIDS, herpes, chlamydia. I wonder if we're not raising a generation of celibate women! With the epidemic of sexually transmitted diseases we have been living under, we have to be very careful not to scare our daughters away from intimacy.

JENNIFER | When I was eight years old, I asked my mother where babies came from. She explained and I understood. I had an idea of what it was all about, anyway, but I wasn't exactly sure.

I didn't find the facts frightening because I was too young to care. I really didn't have any feelings, any emotions about it. I was very young.

I got my period last year and I was surprised. I knew what it was about, so I wasn't scared, but I was surprised because I was so young. My mother was thrilled for me. We went out to dinner to celebrate. It was a very important occasion to me.

I can tell my mother anything I want to. She'll listen and we'll talk about it. But I still keep some things to myself. I like my privacy sometimes.

At some point in life, I'd like to get married, but not too fast. I think you should wait until you're grown up. I also don't think you should have sex before you're married. You should wait until you know the person real well. My friends don't have sex with anyone. We know we're too young.

I talk with my mother about lots of things, but birth control is a subject that has never come up. We have talked about divorce, and here's how I feel about it: It's better to stay together and not get divorced. If you got divorced it wouldn't make any sense to get married in the first place.

I feel the same way about abortion: They shouldn't have gotten pregnant in the first place. That's what birth control is for. If someone's gay, it's their life. They can live it their way. It doesn't bother me.

I think it's very important for daughters to discuss sex with their mothers. If you talk to your mother about sex, then you won't learn about it from the wrong people. You can find out what the real facts are from her.

If you learn about sex from other people, you might think there isn't anything wrong with doing it at a very young age.

But I think it's wrong. And so does my mother.

Joanna is forty years old and married. Her daughter, Susan, the oldest of three, is eighteen.

JOANNA | I grew up in an ethnic neighborhood where most of the people were first- and second-generation immigrants from Slavic countries. Nothing about sex was ever discussed in the home. I felt handicapped because of that. What you learned, you learned on the street. I wish I could have talked to my mother.

My growing up made me want very much to have a close relationship with my daughter. But it's very difficult to talk to your daughter about sex. Very early on, it was easy. When she was three, I was pregnant again and tried to answer her questions, but I was very general about it. She asked the next time I was pregnant, too, and this was more specific. But after that she didn't ask a whole lot of questions.

When she was ten, I found it easy explaining to Susan that one day she would get her period. I thought I should tell her at that age because that's when several of my friends got it. I had one friend who had had no conversations at all about it with her mother, and she thought she was bleeding to death. I didn't know too much myself. None of us knew much of anything at that point because we all came from the same background. I wanted my daughter to know.

When Susan started getting involved with boys, around the age of puberty, I think I explained to her what takes place during sexual intercourse. I didn't get down to specifics too much and, once again, she didn't ask a lot of questions. She did confide in me somewhat during her early adolescence and that meant a lot to me.

We have talked about birth control. I'm still of the old school where I very much feel that you don't get involved in sexual intercourse until you're married. I have never had intercourse with anyone but her father and never intend to.

She's been thinking about going to visit one of her boyfriends for the weekend. She's told me about this. I can't advise her anymore, with a yes or a no. I prefer she not go, but I can also understand her feelings. Our closeness is very important to me. I want to keep lines of communication open, all the way through.

I hope that she's not as afraid of having sexual relations as I was. But I'm afraid she really is. She thinks every guy she goes out with is trying to make her. Maybe they are. I tell her that she's at an age where guys are at their sexual prime.

I would like her to be a little more relaxed about sex than I was, but I also want her to have the satisfaction in marriage that I have—to commit herself to one person and to see that a lifetime commitment can mean happiness. I have a wonderful husband and I want her to have one, too.

I guess what I want for Susan is that she fall madly in love, develop an attachment to someone. Instead, she's dating many people and is judgmental. She's setting her standards so high she's not being realistic. She's very upset if boys are not perfect.

I think she's somewhat afraid of marriage. There's such a high divorce rate. I don't want her to feel marriage is such a chancy thing, but I tell her she'll have to work at it as hard as I did. We do agree on abortion: If a baby's not wanted, the woman should abort.

Mother-daughter relationships are so special. Susan is not only my friend, she is almost a reincarnation of me. I see so many things in her that were my feelings when I was young. Through her, I'm reliving a lot of things. We both were ostracized in our neighborhoods because we didn't have the religious beliefs everyone else did. I explained to her I survived those years and they didn't leave any marks on me.

That experience gave me the incentive to become better, more tolerant, more open to other ideas—and I wanted her to have the same feeling. In the long run, she will survive, and those with small minds will remain in their own little worlds.

I love my daughter very much, and I hope that she has a very fulfilling life, much more so than I do, but then again, I can't complain about mine. I'm very fortunate in my marriage, and my husband and I have worked to make it that way.

SUSAN | My mother and I are very close. She sat me down when I was really young, in third or fourth grade and told me the facts of life. That was the initial talk and since then there's been a series of them. She never really explained things in terms of ovaries or testicles. She avoided all the technicalities by showing me pictures in books.

I had known it already and did not learn anything new. It didn't surprise me.

I've always felt I could ask my mother any questions I wanted to. One time I came home from school, I was really young, and saw the word "fucker" on the sidewalk. I asked her what that meant and she told me. Someone at school once talked about rape and I asked her that, too. I was too embarrassed to ask my friends because I didn't want them to know I didn't know.

When I got my period, the first thing she said was welcome to womanhood. I thought, if this is womanhood, it sucks. I didn't want it. We joked about it and she said it meant I could get pregnant but I already knew that. She explained the egg had broken because it wasn't being used, but didn't go too much beyond that. I learned the rest elsewhere, although she always made it quite clear that I was now able to have children.

I didn't ask for a detailed lecture on what was happening to my body and she didn't offer it. I think she sent off for a Kotex kit, which explained all about periods and had the necessary equipment in it.

She talked to me about things like that, but one thing she didn't ever do was put premarital sex in the context of pleasure. If she talked about sex, it was to say you should only have it with your husband or one person. She said to wait for that one person, and with that one person it would be pleasurable.

We used to have wonderful talks at night. She would tell me about her friends from high school, how most of them were married right out of high school and how one of the smartest girls in her class had gotten pregnant and was now working at McDonalds. She grinded it into my brain that this is not something I would want, would I?

Those are the kind of little things that have influenced me. She was trying to tell me to value sex and not to give it away too soon. It had an effect on me then and still does. In terms of marriage, Mother was an "old maid" in her time because she went on to college, which was breaking the rules in her neighborhood.

I don't see myself married for another ten years. Some of my friends are married now and I pity them. I've done a lot of things sexually but not intercourse. I want to hold out for a person I love, though not necessarily someone I want to marry. But I haven't met him yet.

I feel as if I could go to my mother about almost anything and that's a good feeling. As a matter of fact, I've opened her up to the idea of my moving in with someone some day. She joked it off, but she heard me. There is no one I want to do that with, though. I was just breaking ground. She's very conscious of how things look.

Probably the best thing you can do as a mother is to start talking with your daughter when she is very young and make her feel she can come and speak to you. That communication is important. I don't listen to my mother's advice because I'm old enough to make my own decisions. But I feel what is important is letting her know what's on my mind. I don't want to shut her out.

Even if she doesn't agree with me, she's involved nonetheless. We do agree on abortion: I'm pro choice all the way.

Those bedside talks were great, even though, in retrospect, I didn't agree with many of the things she told me. Her main theme was about women who ruined their lives by getting married and getting pregnant too early. But those talks did establish communication for us to talk to each other, to be close in later years.

I always say the reason I act the way I do is that I had all those ridiculous talks slammed into my brain during my formative years. Today, she doesn't have that power over me, but those talks with my mother were one of the greatest things that ever happened to me in my life.

Four mothers were interviewed alone, without their daughters.

Frances, forty-four, has been married twenty-five years. Her daughter is sixteen.

I have never discussed the particulars of sex with my daughter. Never. I tell her, "I trust you." She reads a lot of magazines and learns from hearsay.

I have told her many times that sex is a part of marriage and she has never questioned me further. I was nineteen years old when I was married. I was a virgin. I have no doubt I did the right thing. I walked down that aisle in a white dress and felt proud.

My daughter did not want to be interviewed. She said, "There is nothing to discuss. Sex before marriage is a sin and that's all there is to it. Nobody should get involved in it before then. It's simple: It's a sin."

She shares my belief that when sex is a part of marriage, everything is fine. She knows right from wrong. I've never had to worry about my daughter.

She wasn't allowed to date until she was sixteen, though her friends were dating before then. She's involved with youth groups and group dating. A whole bunch of them go out together. The guys are not boyfriends, they're friends. They go out as friends and the girls pay their own way.

My daughter wants to go to college and has no plans to be involved with anyone, not sexually or romantically. College is the time for learning and for good, clean fun. She knows what other college kids do, but she says it's their business and she'll choose her own friends.

She has gone to church since she was born. We don't pray before meals, but we go to church every week. She has to go. That's where you learn right from wrong.

Church has taught her the same thing: Sex is part of marriage. It says to have enough respect for your own body not to be involved with anyone unless you are very sure of that person and plan to spend the rest of your life with him.

That's why, from her first date, she knew right from wrong. Religious upbringing influences her 100 percent. She wants to walk down that aisle and to belong there. And that's the only kind of guy she'd want to marry, one who wants to marry a virgin.

Mr. Right is going to want a nice girl. That hasn't changed. And everyone knows who's nice and who isn't. She doesn't have any sleazy friends. She'd have to be completely naive to get to her teens and not know there are two types of girls—and two types of guys.

I would have discussed getting her period, but she already knew. And I did warn her about Stranger Danger. I've never discussed childbirth.

We've discussed abortion. I think there are no hard and fast rules. It depends on certain situations and the person involved. My daughter says it doesn't matter what she thinks about abortion because it's nobody's business but the person concerned.

My daughter and I are honest with each other. She can talk to me if there's a problem. Her girlfriends come and talk to me. They ask me to stay when they come over and I start to go upstairs. My daughter says, "Mom, don't feel you have to run away."

I want my daughter to have what I've had: A long marriage. A church wedding. A white dress—and to feel good about it. I want her to have the right inner feeling, and the only way she'll have it is if she is a virgin. The pastor has known her since she was two years old.

I want her to be there and not feel guilty. That's what I want for her.

Patricia, thirty-eight, is married for the second time. Her daughter, Patty, is twenty-one.

I was very young when I was married for the first time and it was to a man who physically abused me. I was a battered wife. He choked me, held me in a corner with a knife and spit at me. He kept telling me it was my fault. I was so young I believed him. There was no way I knew of to get help. So it continued for about a year.

But when I was six months pregnant he beat me especially hard and that is when I left. My daughter has seen her first father only once. She visited him and his wife and Patty heard him beat her stepmother. After that, she never wanted to see him again. My present husband—we've been married for fifteen years and have two sons—is her father, as far as Patty is concerned and she calls him Dad.

Patty started asking questions about her first father when she was only four years old. I didn't know what to say, so I asked the social worker at her day care agency, who gave me good advice. When Patty saw I would answer her questions honestly and openly, her questions started pouring out.

When she was about eight years old, she asked me such questions as, "Do you love my first Dad?"

I answered, "I loved him when you were conceived."

Patty: "But I'm half him and half you and you love me, so you must love him. And if you don't, then you hate the part of me that's him."

My answer: "I love all of you, every part, and always will."

I was very grateful to the social worker, because when it came to explaining the facts of life to my daughter, talking to her about love and sex, it was very difficult. I was advised to tell her that bad things did happen between me and her biological father, but that sometimes things like that happen. I've told her repeatedly her father loves her and so do I. And so does her dad, my present husband.

I didn't want her to think all men beat all women or

that her father is all bad. I think she has learned this. She also has a very strong conviction that if a man ever tried to abuse her in any way, just once, that would be it.

I feel today that Patty is the most together person in our family. She's in touch with her feelings. Still, I'm real careful what I tell her in the area of sex. We have very open kinds of conversations, as much as she wants. Instead of talking about dangerous men, I talk more about caring and loving and the importance of loving men who care about her.

She's now out on her own, working in another city. We're still very close, but I do worry. Patty has never had a [serious] boyfriend, as far as I know. She's beautiful and very bright. She's had lots of boyfriends and lots of crushes, but she's never been able to let go and fall in love. She must have complete control every time.

When she was in high school, I began to worry about her not relating well to men. In college, she told me the other girls in her dorm had a series of boyfriends who stayed over on the weekend. She was always the one who moved out on the weekends because she never had anyone who stayed over. I asked her how she felt about that, if she would like to have a boyfriend stay over. She replied that she wanted to concentrate on her studies and do well. Her roommates used to tell her, "You're the only one who has it together!"

She may be more involved than I know. She knows I worry and she has always been very sensitive. When she started asking how babies are made, I bought her a children's book on the subject. It was illustrated with cutout figures that had no faces. She took the book and drew in faces on the people.

We've talked about rape and she took a self defense course. She says she can take care of herself. And she can. She's sensible. Patty is very concerned that her dad, my husband, love and accept her. It's not always been an easy marriage, but Patty assumes she'll marry and have children someday.

I want Patty to enjoy the intimacy that comes with a good sexual relationship. I believe in the right to abortion. Patty helped a friend get an abortion secretly and told me her friend's mother would disown her if she knew. We've talked about herpes and AIDS. Kids today are going back to traditional ways and are much more careful than we were in the '60s.

Mothers have to start communicating early with daughters and keep it up. But you can't go through their pain for them. They have to do that themselves.

Margarita, forty years old, is married and has three daughters.

My daughters are two years apart; the oldest is seventeen. I never sat them down and told them the facts of life in one sitting. I started early and told a little. As their need to know escalated, I told them more. Now, if there's something they want to know, they come to me and find out.

I was poor, my parents were farmworkers and no one ever told me anything about sex. This was typical in the Hispanic culture. In retrospect, I remember hearing sort of dirty jokes and trying to figure out what they were all about. Mostly, I didn't understand. My daughters learn sex education in school, at least the technical aspects, and they are very straightforward about it.

I didn't grow up that way. There were always those girls who got into trouble and I understood about "not going too far." The '50s was a period of going so far but not all the way. There was a strong double standard between boys and girls, and if girls had a physical need, we weren't supposed to satisfy it. Sex wasn't so much sinful as impractical. It wasn't in a girl's best interest to have sex.

Finally, I did get married and have children and I remember my father looked at me and said, "You're going to be a mother forever. Try to be the best." And I have.

That was the Hispanic way. I'm not so sure that there is a Hispanic way today. It was very traditional, old-fashioned. The reality—of whatever the life your daughter faces today—intrudes. More and more, Hispanics live in cities and that has to change our way of life. It's very difficult for parents to maintain a traditional home today.

I think about my mother's many warnings and sometimes I'm chagrined. Everything she said about not sitting on toilets today is true!

I'm open with my daughters but we don't talk about pleasure and never had a clinical explanation of orgasm.

We have conversations about intercourse, coitus, things like that, but the discussions are somewhat impersonal. They have to be. It's not my embarrassment but theirs. They don't want me to be specific. They're far more comfortable talking in the abstract.

They ask about things going on at a particular moment. There are limitations on both sides, certain inhibitions.

I've discussed birth control with my oldest daughter but not the other two. She has a boyfriend and he is a very nice young man. She thinks he's wonderful. I hope this works out for her not in terms of sex but in happiness and a good relationship. I hope it turns out the best way it can, that she is able to make the best judgments, the least hurtful. I tell her that nothing comes for free.

Mother and daughter relationships have a pattern of their own. Mine is different with each daughter. I try to be patient and let things ebb and flow naturally as far as their need to be close and their need for distance. Everything is easy when they are very young, direct. Now there are corners. I don't lament that. I just note it.

Conversations about periods are different with each of them. About abortion, I say to each of them I'm not certain I would have an abortion, but I'm pro choice.

My relationships with my daughters change frequently, especially in discussions about sex. If one goes away from me, she'll come back. Everything with the oldest is new and harder for me in talking about sex. Then it gets easier.

Charlotte, thirty-five, is married and has a daughter, fifteen.

I was twenty years old in 1971 and abortions were still illegal. To get an abortion you had to be very rich, but even then, I heard stories of women dying from butchered abortions in back alleys. My friends and I were all terrified of getting pregnant without being married. We knew it would be the end.

In the working class neighborhood I grew up in, there were two kinds of girls and that's all there was to it. My parents, especially my mother, warned me that men wanted only one thing and if I gave in and got into trouble, not to come to her for help. My father warned my sisters and my brothers, too—though he was easier on my brothers—that getting pregnant or getting someone else pregnant would be the end of the dreams he had for each of us to get a college education, a good job and a start in life.

Nonetheless, my brothers, sisters and I had active sex lives fairly early. My brothers and sisters never got caught. But eventually, I did, and the nightmare I had grown up with, the prophecies of the worst thing that could ever happen to a girl, happened to me.

I was supposedly the smartest in the family, the one everyone had such big hopes for. I won a scholarship to college and in my senior year I got pregnant. It's a wonder I didn't get pregnant long before then.

I started sleeping with guys when I was seventeen. My parents had warned me that sex was the only thing boys wanted, so I wasn't prepared for the fact that I would want it, too. No one ever told me the facts of life, though in a big family you pick them up fairly young. But no one ever suggested to me that my hormones might be raging, too.

My reaction to the first boy I let kiss me, when I was seventeen, was overwhelming. I must have scared that guy to death. And I wanted more. I also knew nothing about birth control. When I started having sex, went all the way, which was shortly after that first kiss, I didn't use anything and neither did he. I wouldn't have known what to use and he didn't offer to. We just had sex. And I had a lot of sex with a lot of different guys. I douched secretly afterwards and somehow didn't get pregnant.

The irony is that I didn't get pregnant until I fell in love with Jack and had a long-term relationship with him.

Jack was out of college and had a good job and a bright future. He came from an affluent family and my parents warned me about him, that he couldn't be serious about me because his parents lived on a big suburban estate and I lived in a little row house in the city. But he was attracted to me from the first moment he saw me at a party. He came right after and got me. I wasn't a victim, though. I wanted him as much as he wanted me.

He had his own apartment in the city and we always went there and had passionate sex. About three months after this—we used no birth control, although we were both old enough to know better—I missed my period. Then I spotted blood. Then I became terrified. I don't know why I was so shocked. What did I expect to happen?

I went to a doctor and gave a false name. Jack gave me the money. I called for the results of the test. I was pregnant. I told Jack and he became cold and distant. I thought I would faint. He said he did not love me, would not marry me and did not want a baby. Then he became angry and blamed me for everything. Why hadn't I been more careful? And—even though we'd been together day and night for months—how did he know it was his baby? He called me a cheap slut.

I became hysterical. I threw myself on the floor and screamed and cried and raged. What was I to do? Jack said there was a solution. I would have to get an abortion. He would pay. And, he said, I wouldn't miss that much school and could still graduate and get my degree.

"That's an easy solution for you," I yelled. "But what about me? I could die. You'd like that, wouldn't you?"

Jack said he would investigate the situation carefully, lots of girls had abortions and not everybody died. I told him, okay, to find out what he could. He called his friend from college who was then in medical school. The friend came over and spoke to both of us. "It's too dangerous," he said. "Don't do it. I don't know anyone honest who does it. I can't recommend anyone. Get married, have the baby and forget this nonsense."

Jack was depressed. I felt relieved. I loved him and I wanted to marry him. I didn't know how I felt about the baby, because I had never thought of having a baby. Given the circumstances, I absolutely did not want to stay pregnant. If abortions had been legal, I would have had one and felt entirely relieved. But abortions weren't legal.

Jack still did not want to marry me. I was ruined. Disgraced. I couldn't tell my mother, though I wanted to. She'd kill me. I couldn't tell my brothers or sisters—they'd kill Jack. In those days, you didn't threaten law suits, either, because women were in the wrong.

After a few days of threats and pressure, Jack said he would marry me. I was so grateful. We got married, I finished school and I had a healthy baby daughter. He did the right thing by me, but that was the last time he did.

We're still married but Jack made it clear from the beginning he wanted complete freedom. I had no choice. He plays around all the time, I never know where he is and we don't have much of a relationship. It's certainly not a marriage. I am still so frightened about what almost happened to me, I just grin and bear it. Someday, I'll get a divorce. Jack likes things the way they are.

My life is hard, but I have my daughter. I adore her. She is so wonderful, beautiful and supportive. I am strongly pro choice. I remember the fear. But when I think I may have never had my daughter, I feel sheer terror. I love her so much and do not know how I could ever live without her.

We interviewed four daughters on the subject of mother-daughter communications. We did not interview their mothers in order to protect the daughters' confidences and revelations.

Margaret, thirty-eight, is divorced and has two sons.

I'm bisexual and if I had a daughter, I would hope she'd be bisexual, too. In some ways, it's the natural condition. Sexuality is not necessarily linked to reproduction. I'd like my sons to be bisexual, too. I don't like the idea of narrowing my sexual possibilities.

It wasn't until after I was unmarried that I discovered my bisexuality. I like to think of myself as an equal opportunity lover. I haven't had a female lover for more than five years, though. Periodically, I have crushes on women but haven't acted on them recently.

I've had the same male lover for ten years. He is a lover and friend. I can be with either sex comfortably. Men attract me physically and so do women, but in a different way. I feel more comfortable with women sexually, intellectually and socially. I used to think I was a lesbian and too cowardly to admit it, but I really like men, too.

My mother was very loving and very physical. There was a lot of affection in my family, cuddling and stroking and a really sensual way of being together. I had aunts and female cousins, buxom women who drew me to their bodies with big hugs and kisses. In this way, my mother and female relatives let me know that they loved me and that I was very valuable.

I was also strongly attracted to boys. I petted and necked a lot. When I was in high school, I used to make out like crazy on the couch. We did everything we could think of, short of fucking. About that word I just used: I said it when I was in the sixth grade and my mother took me aside and said to me, "That's a filthy word for a very beautiful thing that people do who are married. Don't use that language or think about sex in those words."

When I was nine, my mother told me the facts of life. She talked to me about my body and the change that would take place. I don't know if she recognized the changes that were happening early to me, or if she was just being her usual anxious, compulsive self, which I have become.

I have to give her credit: She didn't talk about orgasms, but she was fairly straightforward in a vague way.

As I got older, I asked more questions. I wanted to know all about sex. My mother couldn't tell me all the details, but she was way ahead of my friends' mothers, who couldn't tell their daughters anything, except to be sure not to get pregnant.

My mother told me about sex in this way: She said first there's the foreplay, and that is for the woman. Then there is the second part, penetration, and that is for the man. That's a practical way to explain things and at the same time to dispel the myth of vaginal and mutual orgasms!

When I knew I was bisexual, I told my mother but not

at first. When I finally did, she was shocked. She accused me of trying to be radical. I told her I wanted to know this woman I really was, and that involved going both ways.

She asked me what lesbians do, that she never knew. I told her, "You remember how you told me the first part, the foreplay, is for the woman and the second part is for the man? Well, there's only the first part." Then I asked her if I had shown any signs of being bisexual when I was growing up. "No," she said, "you were regular."

I was a very active heterosexual when I married at age twenty-one. I had been going with my husband forever. We had a lot of sex and always enjoyed it. Yet, I was always interested in women's bodies. I thought their genitals attractive, their breasts beautiful.

I began to think, what would it be like to have sex with a woman? How does it work? Do I want to do it? After my divorce, I met a woman, far away and safe, and I told her about my ideas. She told me she was having an affair with a woman. I asked her to be my experiment, but it turned out to be a heavy-duty relationship.

What has evolved from my being bisexual is a growing awareness of the possibility of me, an ongoing dialogue with myself, with the person I am growing to be.

Bisexuality is my preference for everyone, though I would not be unhappy if my children were one or the other exclusively. I wouldn't be miserable if they missed out on it. But it's a neat way to be.

It's a richer kind of sexuality and I would not want to go through life not knowing and loving both women and men.

Eleanor, forty-five, is single. She has never been married.

When I was ten years old, I found out that my father wasn't dead. He and my mother had never married. I was playing dress-up and found in the cedar chest letters my mother had written my father but never mailed. They told the whole story of her getting pregnant and his deserting her.

It was obvious they had never married. While it was overwhelming to learn I had been lied to all those years, I actually wasn't too surprised. Despite the fact my mother had told me—but only once—that my father had been killed just before I was born, I don't think I really believed her. It didn't add up: She never talked about him, never told me how they met, never showed me photos of them together, never told me any memories of him and never told me how much he loved the idea that I was to be born.

She had lied to me all along, and it was only to keep up appearances. Even after I found the letters, I couldn't ask her about them. My mother isn't the kind of person you ask anything of. She had such extremes of moods and emotions that I could never approach her. She's the kind of person you try to avoid confronting.

With this in mind, it's obvious my mother and I were not intimate. To this day, we have no communication, though I feel responsible for her and visit her often. I talk to her but she still doesn't talk to me.

Ten was the age I found out about my parents, and ten was the age I got my period. I asked my mother what periods meant, but she never told me. I asked her to get me a book about the facts of life and she said she would. Thirty-five years later, I'm still waiting. My mother did buy me supplies and told me what to do with them but never told me why.

I wasn't frightened when I got my period because I didn't allow myself to have too many emotional reactions at that age. And there wasn't any one to trust or go to if I did get upset. We lived with my grandparents and my aunt, and I knew they were also in on the lie, so I just kept quiet.

I found out about sex from older friends but I didn't hear anything about sex in my home. I picked up bits and pieces and I wasn't always accurate. For the longest time I thought babies exploded out of the belly button. The first pregnant woman I saw scared me because I thought she had a tumor.

You have to understand that everyone in the world knew I was illegitimate, except me. Women blocks away asked me about my last name and if I was related to so and so. When they saw I couldn't answer, they stopped asking.

Sometimes my mother and grandmother would quarrel, and my grandmother would yell at her and tell my mother she was the cause of all the problems in the family. Then they'd both turn on me and scream at me that I had better be perfect and not disgrace the family. They shouted at me that it was up to me to show the world there's nothing wrong with my family. I did it, but at a great price.

I didn't have a sex life until I was graduated from high school, had a job and lived away from home. That was the same year I tracked down my father and went to visit him. I never told my mother, but somehow I think she knows. He had never married and wasn't the least bit interested in me. Ironically, he died soon after my visit, so I only saw him once. But now my mother's story was true: My father was dead. What was still a lie, though, is that they were ever married. Being illegitimate was such a social stigma to me that even after I found him, I told everyone my parents had been divorced before I was born.

I didn't date until I was seventeen. I did a lot of things, but not intercourse. My mother used to check that I got my period on time. She was afraid I'd be like her.

I wanted to get married and have a family, but I've worked so hard to become outstanding in my field, that I didn't have time to develop lasting relationships—though I have been involved with several nice men over the years.

If I had a daughter, I'd answer all her questions. If you're old enough to ask questions, you're old enough to get answers. And I'd give her a box of condoms and tell her to carry them with her everywhere. Today, sex is dangerous.

Having almost been the victim of abortion, I'm not in favor of it philosophically. I was an unwanted child and I'm very happy to be alive. To this day, my mother hasn't told me the true story. Still, my mother never went on welfare and never begged for anything. She worked hard to support me.

I wish I could please her. I wish I could be good enough for her. That's the worst thing: Not ever being good enough.

Sallie, age thirty-three, is married and has two children.

I grew up in a small town where everyone talked about how bad sex is yet everyone did it. My father owned a drugstore and so I knew a lot more of what was going on than other people did.

I didn't know everything, though, and when I was seventeen I got pregnant. It was in the summer time and I was away at camp. It wasn't the first time I had sex, it was the first time I was pregnant. My boyfriend was real mad at me and said I had to do something right away. We were both counselors and took off for the weekend. We found someone who "always took care of the girls at the camp" and made an appointment for the next weekend.

I had an illegal abortion. My boyfriend and I both paid for it. I had no mixed feelings: I didn't want to have a baby and I was absolutely relieved. But I did want to talk to my mother about it. It was awful not being able to.

My mother tells everyone how close we are, but if you don't discuss anything about sex when you're growing up, you and your mother are not close. I don't feel badly about

the abortion I had, but I was very young and perhaps not only could she have helped me avoid it, it would have been nice to have had her at my side when I needed her.

Nothing was ever mentioned in my house about sex. It still makes me angry to say that. I was an only child and had no sisters or brothers to clue me in. Not knowing anything made me eager to have sex. How else could I ever learn about it? I think that's how I got pregnant: I was much too eager. I didn't even enjoy sex that much, I just wanted to do what was never mentioned and so forbidden.

I married my husband when I was in college. I told him everything. We have two wonderful children, and that's all I want. I had another abortion recently. This one was legal. It was my decision but my husband agreed with me.

I didn't tell my mother about either abortion, although somehow I think she knows. I guess I always think my mother knows everything.

I would have liked to have told her about both. That's what mothers are for. It was even hard for me to tell her I was pregnant with the two children my husband and I wanted. She killed a certain part in me that once was hers. All those secrets! Why? I think it's destructive.

She didn't even tell me about getting my period. I had to learn that from my friends, too, and they weren't always accurate. I don't see how such an important part of life can be shut off.

Sometimes, I think my mother's sex life with my father was so bad she couldn't talk about it. Other times I think she's so sexual she's afraid even to mention the subject for fear it might get out of hand. But I know the truth: She couldn't talk to me about sex, and that has been an enormous barrier between us.

When my kids, especially my daughter, ask me about sex, they get answers. I answer them the same way I answer them when they ask me a question about something going on in the news: straightforward, with the facts. That'll help them make their own decisions in life, and you can't do that without information.

My daughter is ten and my son is eight and they both understand about the danger of AIDS. I mean, they understand intellectually, which is all that's necessary right now. They trust me because they can. They tell me everything. I know that will change soon, but right now our bonds are very strong.

Maybe I should understand my mother comes from a different generation and a different background. She was very poor. I was born very soon after my parents were married. Maybe they *had* to get married and that's what scared her into silence. I don't know. There was another option: She could have talked. I love my mother very much. I just wish we could have been friends.

Nancy, fifty-two, is divorced and has three children.

My mother is in her late seventies but when she was a young woman, she was a highly sexual being. She married several times. She was competitive with me for men when I was around seventeen or eighteen years old.

She was very beautiful and I looked just like her, but I was younger. That made her jealous of me, because she was getting older.

The jealousy and rivalry reached its peak when I was nineteen and still living at home. She married for the third time and lorded it over me. I was very promiscuous; I think I had forty-five lovers in one year.

Her positive attitude toward sex was actually good for me, though, because she was always fairly open, answered all my questions and presented sex as one of the true pleasures in life. Now that we are close and have worked out our relationship—through years of analysis for both of us—I appreciate this part of her.

I asked her when I was seven years old, "How is a baby born?"

She answered, "The man puts it in you."

"Where?"

"You have an egg. It grows inside your stomach. He puts it in with his penis."

"Doesn't it crush you?"

"No, it feels good."

"I'm afraid of it."

"Don't be, it's so many years away. By the time it comes, you'll be ready."

That's pretty wonderful stuff from a woman of her generation. I've told my children about the facts of life in much the same way. And, I'm like my mother in many ways: I've been married four times and so has she.

When she told me about sex, the implication always was that she was an experienced woman. She never indicated she had affairs when I was little. When I was older, she was more open about that.

The sense I got was that sex was enjoyable, a little naughty and a lot of fun. She taught me the world will not come down on you if you sleep with more than one person. But, also from her own experience, she gave me an awful sense that once a man has you sexually, you'll be deserted, that you're vulnerable once you enter that relationship. Unless you can snap your fingers and jump out of bed, you are open to being hurt and emotionally injured.

I think that was good advice, too, and really amazing stuff for a mother to tell a daughter. My girlfriends never heard anything like that from their mothers, and I'm grateful my mother and I could talk the way we did and still do.

My mother even said things to me like this: "If you ever get pregnant, you can come to me. You are not alone in this world."

I never talked too much with my girlfriends about my own sexual experiences because I didn't have to. I had my mother. When I was sixteen, she began assuming I was having affairs. If I went out with someone once, she made the assumption we were sleeping together. That really annoyed me because it wasn't always true. Once, when I was twenty-one, a man invited me to visit him for a weekend and she bought me a beautiful sheer robe to wear.

We've gone over these things a million times, my mother and I. What was she trying to tell me about sex? About her? About me? We disagree on the answers and our problems will never be buried, but we've been able to make our peace. She has gotten more and more maternal as she's gotten older and the support she gives me—though sometimes it's mixed—is so wonderful.

I love my mother very much and our closeness has been a big part of my life. She's been there for me through my marriages, divorces and heartaches. The positives are that what she told me about sex was intelligent, well-thought out and ahead of her time. I got the very best in sexual communication, which allows me to do the same with my children.

The negatives were, I think, a factor of the times we lived in. The jealousy and rivalry, though, were very destructive to me, though I now understand it.

If mothers and daughters can talk, they're lucky, as I was. I think it's a gift from mother to daughter when you can grow up and not worry about sex or what it's all about. It frees you to grow naturally and to be at peace with yourself as you grow older.

And that's a big one!

GROWING UP:
MENSTRUATION, DATING AND ADOLESCENCE

MOTHER | For weeks before I got my period at the somewhat late age of fourteen, I thought I had worms: White mucous discharge, which I saw in my hysteria as actually alive and moving, came out of my vagina. I was so frightened I even told my parents about it, though I knew that the vagina was a part of my body I should never mention to either of them.

They were both extremely kind, understanding—and equally uninformed. Also frightened, they took me to the family physician, appropriately named Dr. Wise.

For the first time in my life, my parents left me alone with the doctor, who knew me since I was a baby. I think that in talking to the doctor over the phone he gave them an idea of what was happening to me and that he would reassure me. He examined my breasts—small, swollen mounds—and pointed out to me I had a few pubic hairs, an observation I had already made myself. And then he told me to get dressed.

Safely clothed, I went into his conference room. I felt very important without knowing why. He called my parents in and told me in their presence that the discharge was not worms, it was a signal I would soon get my period.

"You're growing up so nicely!" he smiled, and hugged me warmly. "Your mother will tell you all about it."

I was relieved and even felt reluctantly proud to inhabit a body that manufactured what still looked to me like worms. A few weeks later, the flow of blood began, but my mother did not tell me anything. Neither did my sisters. Despite the silence, I felt it was a time of celebration, a reflection of Dr. Wise's attitude.

I rushed from the bathroom on the second floor of our row house to the basement, where my mother was patiently washing the clothes and putting them through the wringer.

"It's here! I have it! Look!" I yelled in my usually ebullient manner, waving my underpants at her.

"Shh!" she warned me. "The neighbors can hear everything."

She kept on with her work but seemed pained, upset. "You have everything you need? You know what to do?"

"Oh, yes," I enthused. "I'm okay."

She said nothing for awhile but kept staring at me with what I thought was pity. She seemed to want to tell me something, but what it was I still wonder. Instead, she offered me the kind of nurturing she felt comfortable with.

"Give me the pants, I'll wash them," she said. "Go take care of yourself." And she went back to her work.

I immediately telephoned my friends and bragged to them about my new status as a woman. I had mild cramps but wasn't too uncomfortable, so I took three buses to my best friend's house to celebrate. She had gotten her period when she was eleven and didn't quite see what I was carrying on about, but we celebrated with major homemade sundaes. Her mother, grandmother and aunt—my friend had an extended family under one roof—told me how wonderful I was.

It was enough for me. I felt proud. Still, no one explained the connection between menstruation and having babies.

I learned to recognize the signs that meant my period was coming, that I was "falling off the roof," or, more simply "off." I was athletic and involved in my school's volleyball, basketball, baseball and field hockey teams. Sports kept me in shape and I rarely suffered from my period—and rarely stopped doing anything I had already planned to do.

Our gym teachers encouraged us—our gym classes were segregated by gender—to take gym no matter how we felt. No one made much of a fuss about menstruation. But still, no one mentioned what it really meant biologically.

I knew about sanitary napkins but not about tampons. I suffered greatly as a child when I was the one sent to the drugstore and had to buy sanitary napkins for my mother. I had finally decided to be brave about it, but I ran in and out so fast I never noticed alternate supplies.

One day in high school, when I was sixteen, my friend Jack pointed out something thrown on the street. I thought it was a dead rat and screamed. Jack patiently explained to me it was a tampon and how it was used. My ignorance about tampons led him to tell me the facts of life I needed so badly to know.

I immediately bought some tampons and hid them in my bureau. Unfortunately, Jack had not told me every detail: I tried to insert the tampon without removing the cellophane wrapper. My screams of pain brought my sisters to my aid. They were impressed at my daring—they had never used tampons. They suggested if I was going to continue to use tampons—which everyone knew you only used when you were no longer a virgin—that I unwrap them first.

With this kind of background, it's easy to understand my firm resolve that my daughter would be prepared for her period and understand what it meant. When she was ten, I began reading about menstruation with her from *Our Bodies, Ourselves*. She had given the book to me as a gift, and we both became so enthralled by its forthrightness we began to refer to it as *Our Bodies, Our Very Selves*. When something came up in our discussions we didn't understand, we ran to check it out in The Book.

I was more eager to tell Cathy about menstruation than she was to listen, but then, it was never talked about in my home and she heard it all the time. I told her how exciting it would be when she got her period. I wanted to make sure she felt good about herself and her gender.

At age twelve, when fuzz began to appear on her legs, I told Cathy not to shave her legs. "You're lucky you don't need to shave your legs because you have such fine, blonde hair," I told her. "Once you shave, you always have to shave, because it grows back darker and coarser. So don't do it."

The next day she shaved her legs.

Cathy liked to hear the history and mythology of menstruation more than the facts that might apply directly to her. She was fascinated when I told her some American Indian and African tribes relegated women to special tents or huts during their periods so that their bleeding wouldn't cause bad things to happen. Though they were banished by men, other women celebrated these women and their power.

We talked about religions that classify menstruating women as unclean. We talked about the view among some women that monthly bleeding is an affliction, a curse, another burden women have to bear.

"But it you don't want to be pregnant, the nicest feeling in the world is that of menstrual cramps!" I pointed out.

I wanted Cathy to have a positive attitude toward the wonders of her body, not shame. When boys have erections, they look upon them with pride. Girls get the message from society and many religions that their bodies are dirty or evil. If we don't like our bodies, we can't possibly like ourselves.

One of the top concerns of pre-teens and teenagers is

menstruation—in addition to wet dreams, masturbation, homosexuality, intercourse, pregnancy, birth control and sexual diseases. But menstruation can't be honestly discussed if it's taken out of the context of the young girl's emerging sexuality. That's why the how-to books, pamphlets and school lectures are distorted if they only discuss what happens to the ovary, what kind of sanitary supplies to use and what medication to take for cramps. Now is the time for an open discussion of sex.

A friend tells me that when she was eight years old, her mother told her she'd grow hair and bleed soon. My friend expected to bleed from her armpits!

When Cathy got her period at age thirteen, she was prepared if not entirely overjoyed. Her brothers and I celebrated her coming of age with a gift and dinner out. She had some discomfort but she understood getting her period was a momentous occasion, a rite of passage that merited celebration and honor.

Mothers can make daughters feel proud of their biology, despite the negative message of our chauvinistic society. Judith Arcana, an honest and caring observer of parent-child relationships, has written an instructive story on menstruation called *Celebrating Rachel: A Book for Daughters and Mothers*. In it, Rachel's mother talks about her connection to other women. She tells Rachel, who, at age twelve, has begun to menstruate,

> . . . I see the menstrual cycle as a bond among us. Our blood is a symbol of our lives, linking all women everywhere, back through time and across the world. Menstruation is . . . one of the things special about

being a woman: The blood of life flows through our bodies. Because we live in a time when our beauty and power are not recognized, it's hard to feel good about being female.

At the very moment I felt strong bonds to my daughter, she pulled sharply away from me. When she was fourteen, she almost totally shut me out. Cathy had lots of secrets and few questions. When she wasn't belligerent, she was distant. I felt the loss of her friendship and wonderful humor. I could only wait to get her back again, not the old Cathy but the new one, the young woman.

Her rejection of me coincided with an active interest in boys and close relationships with her girlfriends. She still didn't date but started going to parties, informal get togethers at friends' homes.

Her "formal" social life began in sixth grade with a dancing class, by invitation only. I was appalled at its irrelevancy, that some of her friends were excluded and that classes would reinforce sexual stereotypes of "ladies" and "gentlemen." Cathy insisted on going and I paid the fees with many misgivings. But I was furious when I learned she had to wear a high-necked dress and white gloves.

"White gloves!" I raged. "Are they crazy? That's antediluvian. I will not buy white gloves."

A friend of mine, from nursery school carpool days, heard of my protests. "Don't worry," she told me, "I'll get Cathy a pair of white gloves. Just let her go to the series."

I relented, and the night of the first dance, my friend showed up with a pair of white gloves—white garden gloves. Cathy laughed. We agreed the gloves put it all in proper perspective.

Even when we weren't communicating, we still communicated. But I still remember Cathy's apparent anger at me when she was fourteen, her first year of high school. We came back together again—this time as one adult and one adolescent, instead of one adult and one child—when Cathy got mononucleosis. Those two months at home, at the end of which she switched schools, gave us a chance to talk quietly and calmly: Neither of us could go anywhere.

Katharine Hepburn has described the state of the nation's psyche as somewhat suspect today. "How happy are people?" she asked in an article in *Family Circle* magazine. "It seems to me that the world is rapidly becoming a very peculiar place. People are just glutted with desire . . ."

I believe there is a difference between sex education and sex, a difference between telling a young woman how wonderful romance is and forcing her into a prescribed role in society. Cathy and I talked about our lives in those days of her sickness and it was healing to both of us.

I told her how I had worried as a teenager that I would not have a weekend date and how harmful that pressure is. I described how my family pressured me to find a man. I told her about the time I was sixteen and had a date for a dance. I had worked after school in a toy shop and saved enough money to buy a pair of black high heels with straps. I bought them on a Saturday and when I came home from school on Monday, I went to my closet to try them on. They weren't there. In their place was a pair of Capezios, flat black shoes.

In shock, I ran to my mother. What happened to my shoes? She explained she had gone into town and exchanged them. I would be too tall in high heels. After all, I was five feet-six inches.

I was stunned. My mother was afraid to go out of the house. She never went shopping with me. But it was so important to her for me to be shorter than any man—even one she hadn't met yet—that she fought off her agoraphobia and returned my high heel shoes. The message was clear: Women do not create any problems or embarrassments for men. Men are more important than women. I was crushed. I wore the Capezios.

I told Cathy it's important for women to have other options beside marriage. I was so hurt by my parents' intense need for their daughters to marry—to be safe in their terms—that I never asked Cathy about any of her boyfriends.

This led to another one of our famous misunderstandings, one that wasn't cleared up until we worked together on this book. Cathy tells me she always thought I didn't care if she dated or not just because I didn't ask her if she had boyfriends. The truth was I didn't want her ever to think her value was based on her ability to attract men.

Actually, I deeply wanted her to be "popular," to have boyfriends, to have fun. I had discarded my parents' values but only to a point: It meant a great deal to me that my daughter love and be loved, but I didn't burden her with my needs—even though I wanted to! And I am truly and honestly delighted that she is five feet-nine inches—and beautiful.

As Cathy began to date, we began to talk about relationships. Marilyn Machlowitz, a writer and consultant,
describes a relationship as "that murky area between a one-
night stand and marriage." My daughter and I were not
sophisticated enough to look at it that way, but we did man-
age to discuss the spectre of teenage pregnancy. We talked
in the abstract. She never mentioned her friends. I never
mentioned mine. But we understood one another.

I, of course, was divorced and was dating. It amused
me somewhat when the young son of a man I frequently
saw became enamored of Cathy and asked her out. He had
no wheels—only his father's car. I remember the night
when my friend and I drove his son and my daughter into
town to see a concert. We picked them up later and had dinner together.

I remember thinking, "Is this what I've worked so hard
to achieve these past few years—to double date with my
daughter?" I included Cathy whenever I could on vaca-
tions, dates, assignments, because she and my sons are
more fun to be with than anyone else in the world.

But double dating? That was more than I could handle,
and we've never done it again. I felt that way, I think,
because I was a single woman. I've noticed frequently, and
in my own house, that children want to keep their love lives
to themselves. In their own way, daughters create definite
parameters between their personal lives and those of their
mothers. Daughters want to do their own thing. They want
their mothers to do something else.

Teens, in their need to be like everyone else, want their
parents to be more conservative than they are. I thought

about one of my children's friends who told me, with great disgust—and rightly so, I think—that her parents were always stoned. This youngster had been known to be stoned herself, but she was deeply offended by her parents' misdeeds, or perhaps by their moving into a territory of experimentation that she wanted to reserve for herself.

Because my daughter often tries to protect me from being shocked, especially in matters referring to sex, I smiled to myself as she apologized recently for playing her favorite Jimmy Buffett tape. We listened to a couple numbers and then she said, "Mom, you're not going to like this next one." The next one was, "Why Don't We Get Drunk and Screw?"

I wasn't shocked with the parody of the singles bar scene. I asked Cathy if she thought the word "screw" would offend me? "Of course not," she said patiently. "I thought you'd be offended because it was so sexist." I was wrong again!

Because we know we don't always read each other perfectly, we are very careful of one another's feelings.

The Planned Parenthood book *How to Talk with Your Child about Sexuality* says a top concern of teens is whether menstruation goes on forever. Cathy never asked me about menopause. I remember how my mother suffered, as many women do, and finally had a hysterectomy—one of the most "popular" forms of surgery performed in the United States.

I wondered if it would be the same for me. Recently, my periods stopped and I went through an uncomplicated menopause—no problems, no pain, no estrogen, no hot flashes. I've told Cathy how lucky I was that menopause was as painfree as my periods had been. And my "change of life" involved no overt change of life, except that now I have mammograms each year.

Still, menopause does call for reflection, for putting a period on my period. Recently, I met some friends I hadn't seen for many years. They told me I looked wonderful and then asked if I had "found" anyone yet. I assured them I had found someone. They looked relieved.

"Who have you found?" one of them persisted in asking.

"Me!" I announced. "Me!" Not a bad discovery—for mothers or daughters.

DAUGHTER | Getting your period—I've never used the word "menstruation"—is one of the biggest things that happens to a young girl. It is very hard to understand and to adjust to.

When I first heard from my mother and at school that something inevitable was going to happen to me and it would happen every month for nearly the rest of my life—I said, "No way, this can't be. You're totally wrong. That can never happen to me."

That was my first reaction. Then, my friends began to get their periods and I didn't, so I began wondering when I was going to get it. It was a strange dichotomy: I still didn't want to get my period but then again I was worried I never would.

Once again, because I really didn't want to hear about

it, I didn't listen to my mother's explanations about menstrual cycles. When we were told about it in school, my friends and I didn't pay attention, either. We giggled through each educational film shown to us and took a lot of teasing from the boys in our class, who did not watch along with us.

Even so, I didn't have any real hangups or concerns because my mother seemed very calm about menstruation, and as far as I could see she never curtailed her activities or suffered from cramps or any other problems when she had her period. In many households, the kids are aware that their mother is "unwell" and don't quite understand what's going on. But my mother was lucky—and so were we.

Prepared though I was—unlike my mother—when my period did come at age thirteen I was amazed when it started in my body. My main reaction was: This is something I have no control over. I was in temporary shock.

I thought it was an awful thing. I can't believe it. I want someone to fix it. In retrospect, I agree with the reaction Susan had when she got her period and felt, "It sucks!" (chapter 5).

My mother treated my getting my period as a day of great celebration, and that helped a lot, but it was also slightly embarrassing. I didn't completely understand why she was so thrilled. For a long time, I had asked her for a pair of Dr. Scholl's sandals. She finally got them for me—in honor of my "coming of age."

I've read a lot recently of young girls' being honored when they "become women" with flowers and parties and other salutary rituals. I laugh to think my award was a pair of Dr. Scholl's sandals. Those sandals meant a lot to me when I received them.

Today, I'm accustomed to menstruation. I never felt ashamed of having my period, though I do remember being embarrassed when I was in my early teens and ads for tampons were on television. I felt uncomfortable in front of my brothers and their friends, in a crowd of guys. They never said anything or made fun of me, but I was always uneasy.

However, my cycles aren't as easy as my mother's. Sometimes I get cramps, crave certain foods (especially chocolates!) or get really moody. Some of my friends have severe cramps and tell me that it's awful.

I make sure I have complete gynecological checkups at least once a year so I know I'm really okay. Before I went away to college, my mother made appointments for me, but at age eighteen I realized it was time for me to take responsibility for myself. That's an important part of growing up, of being a woman instead of a little girl.

Some doctors prescribe medication such as Motrin or Anaprox to relieve the symptoms of dysmennorhea. But I don't know if drugs are the only answer. It's not that I'd rather suffer or have other women suffer. It's that I don't like what some of my friends have told me about the side effects of the drugs. I feel very strongly that drugs are not the only solution to medical problems and that all medications should be used sparingly. My friends tell me some drugs for menstrual problems relieve the pain but also knock them out, make them dizzy and leave them with a general sense of disorientation. Women need to be aware of the effect caffeine, sugar and alcohol can have on their bodies at varying times in their monthly cycle.

There is a difference between people with serious health problems getting necessary relief from drugs and people with doctors who liberally prescribe drugs for every ailment. Recently, I went to an ear specialist because I had an earache. He thought that perhaps it was from grinding my teeth at night—I was in the middle of finals. He advised me to take Valium every night to see if the pain stopped.

When I refused to take drugs for this minor problem, he was upset. He accused me of questioning his judgment. He was right! I was! I can see why women cave in and often blindly obey their doctors, but it's always a good idea to find out all you can about your problem and make your own decision about taking medication. For menstrual problems, my decision is not to.

Maybe if my discomfort during my periods were worse, I would change my mind about medication. As it is, I feel I can handle it.

Menstrual pain used to be dismissed as "female complaints" and classified as imaginary. The wonderful book, *Our Bodies, Ourselves,* did a lot to help women understand this is another area where it's not our fault. I often refer to *Our Bodies* to read about menstruation, premenstrual syndrome, endometriosis and toxic shock.

My friends and I knew so much, yet we really knew so little about our bodies' cycles. I remember when I was in the sixth grade, my girlfriends and I used to watch one girl or another and say, "I bet she's getting her period! I bet she has it!" We were really into it.

Sometimes we'd look for clues. We used to notice when girls wore skirts every day for a week instead of jeans. We thought that meant something. What it was supposed to mean I don't really know, but we would speculate about it.

One thing some of my friends used to mention was how their mothers suffered when they had their periods. I never heard one complaint from my mother. Never.

A lot of the stuff they showed us in school about menstruation was women in discomfort. Or we'd be reading about some ancient or foreign culture and there'd be a sentence about how women who menstruated were banished from the rest of the group, or weren't allowed to touch food, or brought bad luck. I couldn't equate that with anything that went on in my life or my mother's. I remember saying at that time, "My mother doesn't have that! She couldn't possibly or I would know about it."

My mother never gave me negative feelings about menstruation, but I kept getting negative messages from others. After awhile, I did accept it, but at first I said, "No way." It sounded like the most inconvenient, messy thing I ever heard of.

One day, when I was fifteen, a free sample of Playtex tampons came in the mail for my mother. I had just read an article about how dangerous the chemicals were that were used in Playtex tampons. I couldn't believe we got a free sample in the mail. Also, my mother had always warned me never to use anything that comes in the mail, except maybe laundry detergent. She told me to throw everything else away.

I told her not to use the tampons because they could be

dangerous. She translated that to mean I thought all tampons were dangerous, and later, when stories came out for the first time about the relationship between the use of tampons and of toxic shock, she told everyone that I had known about it all along, long before anyone else!

She kept coming back to me, saying, "Okay, Cathy, what else do you know? You can tell me."

I didn't know anything, but I learned a lot about my body and wasn't afraid to ask questions, even if sometimes I didn't like the answers. I was not afraid to learn and I still can't think of anything to be afraid of connected with getting my period or anything else about the biological facts of life.

I went through cycles about getting my period: First, my friends and I were worried. Then we were excited because we couldn't believe it would really happen to us. Then we got it and thought it was fairly inconvenient. Finally, we got used to it.

But I have to admit that today many of my friends in college are relieved when they get their periods.

As an adolescent, I had a great feeling of wonderment about what was happening to my body. It was scary and it was wonderful.

Along with the hormonal changes came emotional ones. I began to be very interested in boys. I wanted to go to parties, to date, to be grown up, to be independent. Many of my feelings were influenced by my mother's attitudes and opinions, but I wanted to form my *own*, to escape her close supervision.

I felt very grown up. I was positive that I knew what

was best for me. I fought to be my own person, which is an important part of growing up. On the other hand, my head was filled with the passion and intensity of Edna St. Vincent Millay and Emily Dickinson, whose poems had been read to me as nursery rhymes. I was an incurable romantic! It's a wonder I got through those years. Or that my mother did.

My early teens were the time I finally had a lot of questions I wanted to ask about sex, except I didn't want to ask my mother about them. I knew she'd answer, but I was trying to distance myself from her. When kids ask about sex, they deserve answers, but it was apparent to me that my friends who did ask weren't getting the facts.

It's not so much specifics we all wanted to know. We wondered if we were normal, like everyone else. Would we ever get curves? There were other questions, too. When should we start dating? What should we do on a date?

I was already somewhat experienced in that area. When I was in second grade, a neighbor, Paul, who was in my class, asked me to go to the movies. My mother said I could go with him, and he and his father showed up at my house to take me. I was excited—so excited that I wasn't let down when the projector broke in the middle of the movie. We left without seeing the end of it. I like to think that mishap helped prepare me for other dates I've had!

My girlfriends and I had special boyfriends, even if the boys didn't know about it. We talked about "going" with certain boys; that meant we talked to them a lot every day in school. And, we had crushes. Lots of them.

When I was fourteen, the son of a man my mother was

dating asked me out. The son was sixteen and very nice but I never took him seriously. I thought it was a game we were playing, double dating with my mom and his dad, sort of a situation comedy show, with life imitating art. I also knew my mother wasn't thrilled by the idea, although she liked him and his father very much.

When I realized how serious the son was about me, I backed out. If it was a game I was playing, it was a dumb one. Perhaps if I had a crush on him, it would have been fun. But even then, I doubt if I could have handled it. I *wanted* to care more than I did, but I didn't. It's not an awful thing—to double date with your mother—if you can handle it. But for me, it was the wrong person.

I liked boys but never made much of a fuss about them in front of my mother. She asked about them but never made me feel that I had to have a date or had to have a boyfriend. She was low-key about the whole thing and her attitude made it easy for me to decide to go to a dance with my girlfriends, if I wanted to, rather than with a boy; or, to include my girlfriends when a boy invited me to go somewhere with him; or, simply, to spend the evening with my girlfriends or just be alone.

The pressure she felt growing up, to grab the first man who would marry her, is totally absent from my life. Yet, for many years, I thought my mother didn't want me to have a boyfriend, that she thought it would be better not to be involved with anyone. Writing this book, I learned for the first time she didn't feel that way at all—she just didn't want to lay the whole dating trip on me because it had given her so much anxiety as a teenager.

I know I've benefited from not having it drilled into my head that I had to have a boyfriend at all times and that my goal in life should be to get engaged and married. Right now, I'm busy in law school and it's hard to find time for a social life. However, I know it is important for me to have someone in my life whom I care about because it balances out everything else.

Growing up is hard to do, as the song (paraphrased) goes, and I certainly found it that way, even though I was lucky to have an understanding mother. But mothers can't do it for you, you have to go through it yourself. All they can do is try to guide you. All daughters can do is try to listen to their advice.

The nicest part is when you can calmly look back on those adolescent years—the ups and downs, the insecurities, the love-hate relationship with your mother, the astounding changes in your body—and realize how amazing the whole process was.

Another nice part: To look back and realize that your mother was right about a lot of things—and that you don't mind a bit.

THE NITTY GRITTY:
TEENAGE SEX, HOMOSEXUALITY, AIDS, AND AN OLD-FASHIONED IDEA, COMMITMENT

MOTHER | Many mothers tell me they would hate to be young women growing up in today's confusing world of sexual relations, as their daughters—and mine—are doing. Sex today has Alice in Wonderland qualities: Things are seldom what they seem. "I could never pick my way through the maze of accepted sexual practices and the taboos," one woman says. "The world of dating and mating has different rules from when I was growing up, but many of the controlling factors—such as we are still the ones who get pregnant—have not changed."

I agree. Between my coming of age and that of my daughter's, there was a major sociological upheaval called the sexual revolution. This in no way made women equal with men, especially in that major target of the revolution:

bed. Despite the sexual revolution, the Pill and the legalization of abortion (I'm ambivalent about the first of these, concerned about the second and strongly in favor of the third)—things still are not equal.

In fact, in the area of the bedroom, things often seem less than equal, with men literally remaining on top.

My daughter understands this inequality, though I have found it painful to explain to her that the kind of romance depicted in the media and in contemporary music can easily mean an unplanned pregnancy, sexually-transmitted diseases and even death, not just from Acquired Immune Deficiency Syndrome (AIDS), but also from birth control pills and intrauterine devices. And then, if you live, there's the emotional trauma of romance when it's over, the vulnerability, the depression. Despite the sexual revolution, when an affair ends, it still hurts.

I sometimes wonder if being sexually active is worth the many risks it has today, but then, I'm a grown woman whose hormones have calmed down a bit. For younger women faced with so many choices and so many consequences, wise decisions can only be made by asking a lot of questions and finding out answers. That's where mothers, brave mothers, can be of help, in providing the backbone, support and nurturing necessary to make such a difficult evaluation.

How different from the way I grew up in the '50s, firmly entrenched in the double standard, with no doubts about "right" or "wrong" or what "nice" girls did or did not do.

The fear of pregnancy was as terrifying to my generation as the fear of AIDS is today. The end result was the same: Our lives were over. Fear of having a child without also having a husband convinced many of us to remain virgins, despite our strong desires and biological and emotional needs for sex. This unrealistic and fragile structure, bolstered by very little information about sex, blew into bits in the '60s with *Bob and Carol and Ted and Alice* sharing a bed, open marriages and wild sexual escapades. The only commandment was: Do what feels good. Women included.

Even though *this* Carol was never a part of the '60s' new sexual scene—I was married and faithful—I was an intrigued observer of single people openly having sex lives, couples living together, mate-swapping and sexually "doing your thing." I learned things about sex I should have always known, and I and other women of my generation realized that we too have sexual yearnings beyond those of procreation.

I also saw that many women were wounded emotionally by the studied lack of commitment or caring. Many women were strewn carelessly in the wake of the explosion of the sexual revolution—and so were many marriages.

When I was divorced in the '70s, a more realistic knowledge of my biological needs helped me survive the double whammy of divorce and once again being single in a world with a diminished double standard—but still most emphatically run by and for men. The latter was an observation shaped by another revolution, the women's movement, which came along in time to nurse me through divorce and raising three small children alone. The women's movement saved my life: I wasn't liberated, I was fired from my job as wife.

In many ways, the '70s were easier to comprehend sexually than today's sexual realities. Frankly, if I were my daughter's age, I would be scared today. Can a kiss, the exchange of saliva, kill you? Are there contraceptives for tongues and lips? If we can be sounding boards for our daughter's concerns, even if we don't have all the answers, we will be contributing in a major way to their lives. And to our own.

Though no one would describe me as moralistic, there is something I feel very strongly about. It's adultery, being unfaithful to your marriage partner. I am against this form of betrayal. When I was first divorced, I said, "I hate married men." They always asked me out. I never went.

These men told the same story: Their wives were frigid, slept in long underwear and always had headaches. They hadn't had sex with their wives for years—despite the fact they also became fathers with regularity. I was insulted by their pleas to sleep with them and didn't believe how irresistible I had become. I had known many of the men for years and they had never shown the least bit of interest in me when I was married or another man's "property." Now I was considered fair game, but it didn't seem fair to me.

My children have long heard my opinion of adultery. If they had any doubts, they were dissipated the day John Belushi died. The story broke late on a Friday afternoon and I was at the newspaper. My kids called to find out if it was true the actor had died. "What did he die of, Mom?" my daughter asked me. My outrageous reply was, "Adultery." What I meant was that if Belushi had been with his wife, he would still be alive. Later revelations of the sad story proved me right, if not about adultery, at least about Belushi.

Today, some adultery is on hold because of the fear of sexually-transmitted diseases. It's not the way I'd like to see that problem resolved, but I'm not unhappy with the results. Having many partners, whether you are single or married, is dangerous today.

The love generation of the '60s has grown up, but it is also true that sexual relations have not sprung back to the point they were impaled on three decades ago. The majority of American women assert their right to an active sex life—if not verbally then by their actions. But a small segment of women now speak openly of the joys of being celibate.

Celibate is a word that was buried by hippies and smothered by multiple orgasms. The idea of celibacy is more than not having sex; it also means not spending every free moment looking for Mr. Right or Somebody-Who-Is-Eligible so you can have sex. Celibate women want to devote their energies elsewhere. Martha Leslie Allen of Washington, founder of a magazine, the *Celibate Woman*, says her readers are not anti-male or anti-sex. Their solution to the problems surrounding an active sexual life are not religious or moral. Being chaste by choice is an option they choose as an answer to our "sex-rife society."

Celibate women say they are free to do other things, free of the anxiety of always looking for *someone*. Many young women, my daughter tells me, remain celibate between long-term relationships. No one-night stands for them.

Celibacy, when observed for a lifetime, is indeed a final solution, but it also eliminates another problem: Sexually-transmitted diseases. Mothers who want to discuss these epidemic and dangerous diseases with their daughters will find authoritative discussion of them in *Our Bodies, Ourselves.*

Of some eighteen diseases associated with sexual activity, the most common are vaginitis, gonorrhea, chlamydia, ureplasma, herpes, syphilis and genital warts. Women often get painful vaginal or yeast infections—and once they are cured often get them again. We have to tell our daughters that not only do they need medical treatment but their sexual partners do, too, or symptoms will continue to return. I've told my daughter about a friend of mine who had a severe yeast infection for almost a year. She was in such pain it was difficult for her to walk. For weeks, her problem was not properly diagnosed or treated. When it finally was, it kept recurring. She eventually learned her partner—a man who had sexual relations with many other women—was reinfecting her.

"The least he could have done is wash," she told me bitterly. It was months before she was physically and emotionally ready to have sex again—with a different man.

Before the specter of AIDS arose to haunt us, genital herpes was the frightening disease of the moment, linked by many to the new sexual freedom and a variety of sexual partners. An estimated seven million to twenty million people have herpes, a disease that includes blister-like sores and lesions on various parts of the body, swollen lymph nodes, fever, painful vaginal discharges and headaches. And that's just the first attack. Although 40 percent of herpes victims never have a second outbreak, the average sufferer, according to Dr. Allan H. Bruckheim, has three or four recurrences a year.

Cures for herpes are often reported, but as yet there are only palliative drugs. Researchers are optimistic about finding a cure in a new and experimental class of antiherpes drugs now being tested on animals. The next step will be tests for their safety and then tests on humans will begin.

The only conclusion I can draw from the dreary list of sexually transmitted diseases is that there is no such thing as casual sex—though I truly wish there were—and that is what I tell my daughter. In a letter published in *Ms.* magazine, Polly P. Starkey of Flagstaff, Arizona, says, "Let's regroup and look at sex as an expression of caring, giving and relating. Only then will we approach sexual freedom."

"Caring, giving and relating." What nice words. How nice it would be to read them more than once to those wonderful folks who bring us prime-time television, where sex is easy, available, without birth control and without consequences. A recently study conducted by Cleveland, Akron and Canton, Ohio affiliates of Planned Parenthood Federation of America in which volunteers viewed 123 hours of television, found the television shows "sexually exploited" their teenage viewers. A New York City study by Planned

Parenthood reports that high school students who watched a lot of television became dissatisfied with their virginity.

The charge is that television encourages teens to have sex by depicting frequent bedhopping in shows like "Dallas" and "Dynasty" without any attempts to teach sex education or contraception. This charge is added to an older one, that television also promotes violence against women and promulgates sexist stereotypes.

When my children were younger, I carefully monitored and rationed their television viewing time. All three were asked to be on a television show about kids watching television and what their favorite shows were. Cathy made quite a stir when she announced, "My mother won't let us watch anything violent on television, like the news or commercials."

A national survey of teenagers suggests that more than half of all seventeen year olds are sexually active and that only one-third of sexually active adolescents use contraceptives on a consistent basis. The United States has the highest teen pregnancy rate among industrialized nations, with 1.1 million adolescents becoming pregnant each year.

Another report—it's obvious that teenage sexuality is the latest activity to come under public scrutiny—by the prestigious National Academy of Science showed that most teenage mothers drop out of school, are more likely to be unemployed and that their babies run disproportionate risks of dying in infancy or becoming teenage mothers themselves. Yet, wearing blinders, the Reagan administration loudly opposed the reports' suggestions to give contraceptives to teenagers and to maintain school-based health clinics.

In Chicago, the Du Sable high school's clinic treats teenagers for general health problems, including dispensing birth control information and devices. The year before the clinic was opened in 1985, three hundred of the school's one thousand female students had been pregnant. No students are seen by the clinic without parental permission. Anti-choice adults have picketed the clinic and tried to shut it down. At public hearings, the comment of one student, a mother at age fifteen, moved me deeply. She asked critics of the clinic: "Where were you when we needed you?"

I sympathize with mothers who don't want to talk about unplanned pregnancies, but the frightening statistics force us to speak up, and, I hope, in a nonjudgmental way. Many mothers naively believe—choose one—that their daughters know nothing about sex or know everything. Neither is true.

I'm aware from recent conversations with my daughter that she simply tuned out many of the important facts about sex that I told her. If she had been listening, how could she think you get pregnant only when you have your period, despite the logic of how she came to that conclusion? (See chapter 4.) Mothers have to talk to their daughters and keep talking. There's a lot more to sex education than the anatomical differences between girl birds and bees and boy birds and bees. It's a process that mothers can set in motion.

We deceive ourselves if we think our daughters are

asexual. Florence Aadland, mother of Beverly Aadland who had an affair—others would call what happened statutory rape—with Errol Flynn that began when Beverly was fifteen, leans on an old bromide when she says: "My baby was a virgin . . . I ought to know. I'm her mother and she told me everything."

Oh, yeah?

I speak up about unplanned pregnancies because I'm battling an enormous superstructure that profits from teenage sexuality. Some celebrities work against sexual sanity. They're formidable foes, especially Madonna, who had a hit song that idealized teenage pregnancy and adolescent single mothers. Her video, "Papa Don't Preach," is as appalling to writer Ellen Goodman as it is to me.

Goodman calls the song "a commercial for teenage pregnancy." It's about a teen who is pregnant, decides to keep her baby and begs her father not to preach because everything is going to work out well. "The happily-ever-after image has about as much to do with the reality of adolescent motherhood as Madonna's figure has to do with pregnancy," Goodman writes. "It's artificially inseminated with romance." The writer adds: "Adolescents are fed the pop image of a love that is zipless and parenthood that comes without bills or diapers."

Perhaps teen sex is due to hormones or to a quest for intimacy and affection. Whatever we think ,the grim statistics indicate the importance of initiating an ongoing dialogue with our daughters in order to discuss the realities —as well as the romance—of sex.

Among the many sexual matters never mentioned

when I was growing up was sexual identity. According to the American Association for Marriage and Family Therapy, at least one in ten teenagers has difficulty with sexual identity. They don't know what these ambivalent feelings mean and often fear being "found out" if their attractions during adolescence are not straight, socially-acceptable heterosexuality. If daughters can discuss these problems with their mothers, being able to accept themselves will be that much easier.

Family therapists describe our sexual feelings as "preferences." Psychologists and psychiatrists are the same folks who for years classified and treated homosexuality as a mental illness. I consider people's sexual choices as "orientation," not "preference." I can't imagine anyone in our self-righteously heterosexual society choosing to be homosexual. I believe it's biologically ordained.

To condemn homosexuality is bigoted and unfair, I tell my daughter. My general attitude toward other people's sex lives also extends to homosexuality: People have the right to do whatever they want in the privacy of their bedrooms. I just don't want to know about it. I'm not interested.

I openly discuss with my daughter women's liberation, the sexual revolution and gay liberation. Bisexual and homosexual women and men are organizing to protect their rights. The recent U.S. Supreme Court decision making sodomy and oral intercourse between homosexuals illegal is a flagrant infringement on the right to privacy. I believe that decision was made by a conservative court to lay the groundwork to invalidate the right to abortion, which is based on the Constitutional right to privacy. However, I also know our homophobic society may also enact repressive laws under the guise of protecting society from AIDS.

My daughter—and sons, too—learned about homosexuality when they were toddlers. I told them that some people are attracted to their own sex or to both sexes, and there is nothing wrong with that. They brought home from school the words "faggot" and "dyke" and quickly heard my disapproval of phrases that denigrate people. In explaining why these words offend me, my kids learned that I respect the right of consenting adults to have sex with whomever they want.

When I was a kid, I had no idea what homosexuality was, so it's not surprising that I'm still somewhat naive about it.

My innocence is not feigned. I never think anyone might be homosexual because I don't think about people's sex lives. I have to be told. I have known two wonderful single women for many years. They live together and have a warm affection for one another. Fine. I never thought twice about it. I was brought up to think twice about a single woman and a single man living together.

Recently, they told me they are lovers. They wanted to share their joy with me and knew I'd be happy for them. I am. I wasn't shocked, I just had no idea. They've been together longer than most people stay married. And neither of them fears getting a sexually-transmitted disease because they are faithful to one another. As Gretchen says in chapter 5, "the safest person to have sex with is a lesbian who is not an intravenous drug user."

My children and I know a male homosexual couple who have also been together for many years. They tell us of their love and devotion. I think we were uncomfortable at first but we like and respect them both, see their happiness and accept their choices. We also know that in the days before AIDS changed our sexual lives, not all male homosexuals were committed or monogamous. AIDS has changed that, too.

The fear of AIDs has changed many things in our society. One is that mothers who are reluctant to discuss sex—let alone sexually-transmitted diseases—with their daughters are learning all they can about this new plague to discuss its implications with their daughters. Women who avoid the subject of sex because they feel awkward about it are now vocal because of their justifiable fear of AIDS.

The obvious need to be informed so we and our loved ones can survive may also bring about changes in public attitudes toward sex education. No longer can schools or parents get away with innuendoes about sex. No longer can we afford to be embarrassed about sex education or to object to it because it allegedly encourages sex. No matter how we feel about sex, male homosexuals, bisexuals, heterosexual free love or intravenous drug users, we must know the facts about AIDS and tell them to our children.

"It's not a question of morality," says the Reverend Craig Darling, of the National Council of Churches AIDS Task Force, "it's a public health emergency."

Mothers will have to start talking to their elementary-school-age daughters about AIDS, and lesson number one is that not only homosexuals get it.

Other facts: The National Academy of Sciences predicts that AIDS, a deadly breakdown of the immune system, will cause more than fifty thousand deaths annually in the United States by 1991. There is no known cure for this fatal disease, though intensive efforts are underway to find one. Between six hundred thousand and 1.2 million Americans have been infected with the virus since it was discovered in 1981. It has claimed more than thirteen thousand lives. The sad part about the spread of AIDS is that initially little attention was paid to it, despite warnings, because the public believed only homosexuals would get it.

The disease is still so new that we don't know all the answers. Does everyone who has the virus get the disease? If the virus is in your bloodstream, for how many years can it be transmitted? Are condoms the best protection against AIDS?

Mothers and daughters need to find out answers in addition to chastity and monogamy. Relying on our daughters to abstain from sex before marriage will not protect them from AIDS. I hope my daughter thinks of sex in terms of love, pleasure and commitment, not dangerous diseases and death. But knowledge is power and I want my daughter to be informed so she can make intelligent decisions.

So the sexual revolution ends with a bang and a whimper, defused not by moral platitudes but by disease. Casual sex seems ludicrous, and not at all casual, when you realize you're not just having sex with one person but are vulnerable to all of that person's sexual partners and those sexual partners' sexual partners as well. That makes the bedroom very crowded. The orgiastic approach to sex that we read and sang about for years just isn't as much fun these days.

Another chilling effect on the sexual revolution is that spouses can sue for damages if their mates have a sexually-transmitted disease and don't tell them about it. The New York Supreme Court's Appellate Division recently upheld a lower court order that a man undergo a test for herpes as part of a $1.5 million negligence and fraud suit filed against him by a woman who is now his ex-wife.

Cathy knows I believe much of the sexual revolution was liberating, enlightening and often enjoyable for women. It was destructive in its macho message that women should be available sexually for men, no strings attached. The strings are now attached and they are ropes of commitment, caution and respect. Not fear of pregnancy but fear of disease brings us to a new and more mature era of sexuality.

DAUGHTER | My favorite Edna St. Vincent Millay love poem, "Recuerdo," which my mom read to me when I was young, was written in 1920 and begins, "We were very tired, we were very merry—/We had gone back and forth all night on the ferry." But in 1987, a love poem would more realistically be titled "Ode to AIDS and to the Seventeen Other Sexually-Transmitted Diseases."

The romantic world is filled with dangerous sexual diseases, casual sex and unplanned pregnancies. I wish it were otherwise. I much prefer to look at the world of love with romance-colored glasses and to imagine a knight, white horse and setting sun.

If I didn't realize that sex in the late twentieth century can be perilous from my own observations, friends' experiences, and what I read, I'd surely know it anyway from my mother.

She says, "Cathy, what are you going to do? Even a kiss is dangerous." My mother often goes around the house singing a song from the days when she was growing up—my brothers and I refer to her childhood as "the olden days." She sings, "A kiss on the hand might be quite Continental . . ." We stop her before she gets much further.

I hear so many adults saying, "Thank goodness I'm not a young person today and don't have to deal with today's pattern of love, sex and relationships."

My reaction to much of this is to distance myself from it: I set very high standards for myself regarding the type of man I get involved with. Still, I am not opposed to premarital sex, just to casual sex: To me, there is no such thing. I believe commitment and communication are vital not only to deal with the harsh realities of life today but also for my own emotional security.

My attitude, I believe, is fairly typical of today's American women, especially young women. *Glamour* magazine did a survey recently of more than eight hundred women between the ages of eighteen and sixty-five and the results show that we are growing more liberal in our sexual attitudes—at the very same time that we are worried to death about sexually-transmitted diseases. I was not surprised to learn that 50 percent approve of sex before marriage and that 75 percent think if a single woman wants to have a child and raise it by herself, she should.

Not surprisingly, some 47 percent of single women changed their sexual patterns because of fear of AIDS, from which I infer means they stopped having casual sex. But I was surprised that 18 percent approve of extramarital sex, an increase of 6 percent over the previous year's survey.

When I say I set "high" standards for myself, here's what I mean: I can't have a relationship with a man or continue a relationship if I thought he was also involved with someone else. I simply would have to stop seeing him. And that would be for both physical and emotional reasons.

I protect myself in every way from getting a sexually-transmitted disease. I don't get involved with anyone I don't know very well and certainly would not have sex with anyone I wasn't deeply involved with. Of course, when you're a student in law school, romantic involvements are mostly academic: You're much too busy for them.

Another word connected with relationships means a lot to me. It's "trust." I have to have the trust with him that I have with a very close friend before I will sleep with him. He has to *be* my close friend. In other words, I have to know or to think that I know a man very well as a friend before I will consider a physical relationship.

I guess I'm on the opposite end of the continuum from

many young women who feel okay about sleeping around. From what I've seen and heard, it's not so much sex they want as love. They simply mix up sex and love and hope having sex will bring them love and attention. It may mean attention, but not always love and not always commitment. I know that I, too, mix up love and sex but in the opposite way: The close connection between the two makes me very conservative, very cautious about sex. I pursue love first, sex later.

Long before the advent of AIDS, I felt that there should be no sex without love—love based on friendship and trust. Since this is the standard I use for myself, it's hard *not* to apply it to everyone else. I feel strongly about it, even to the point of being judgmental. I can't help being that way because I've seen so many girls get hurt. I try not to judge girls who are more casual with their bodies than I am, but I often think the word "cheap," to myself. I just can't seem to get around doing that.

It's a strong value judgment, based not only on what I see and feel but on what my male friends tell me. Some of my best male friends are great womanizers—but not with me. They're just my friends. And I've learned a lot from them. I'm often the only woman in their lives with whom they are *only* friends. Their relationship with most other women goes something like this—they sleep with them as soon as possible and then never talk to them again. They look at girls as potential marks—and they tell me that. The whole thing is ironic: They don't respect the women they sleep with, but they *do* respect themselves. It's a weird tradeoff. It's called the Double Standard. It's a game of pursuit and capture. Once the hunt is successful, the game is over.

That's the bad news. The good news is that some of these guys, mostly between the ages of twenty-three and twenty-five, are now starting to tire of the chase, the game. Now, they're beginning to tell me, "Maybe I do want a relationship with just one person, just one girlfriend." But they absolutely would *never* consider a relationship with any of the girls they've slept with so casually. That just killed me the first time I heard that from a male friend! They see those affairs as important for some kind of track record they keep in their minds. Sex is separate from a relationship. It counts only when you're keeping score, which they do.

My male friends know that commitment is important to me. I don't even mean commitment for a lifetime or forever: I'm not quite ready for that. I *do* mean commitment for the length of the relationship—whatever that might be.

I'm glad I can talk with my mother about these things because they're so difficult to sort out. Pre-marital sex is something daughters need to discuss with their mothers, no matter how awkward or embarrassing it may be. In 1987, the median age for first marriages is around 23 for women and 26 for men. The average age for first marriages is higher for women in the '80s than in any other decade previously recorded by the U.S. Census Bureau.

The median age for men who marry was 25.5 the previous year. The fact is that women and men are getting married later. Economics have a lot to do with it. It's been said that most of today's young people will not make more money than their parents do—a reversal in the upward trend that had been taking place in the United States for decades. That's why so many young people live at home—they don't earn enough money to live on their own.

Marriages may be postponed but, usually, an active sex life is not. There's another popular lifestyle that is sort of a halfway house between being single and being married. Today, some 2,220,000 Americans "share living quarters with an unrelated adult of the opposite sex"—the Census Bureau's official way of saying "living with someone you're not married to." That figure is four times what it was in 1970.

The lifestyle you choose is a matter of conscience, I believe—of *your* conscience. However, I always have to laugh at the message in a "Cathy" cartoon strip, by Cathy Guisewite. In it, Cathy and her friends are talking about how to know what's right and wrong. In the next to last cartoon segment, one friend tells her, "Cathy, you have to talk to your conscience, that's the only way." In the last one, Cathy is on the telephone, shouting into the receiver, "Mom!"

My mother isn't my conscience and I'm not hers. But her approval means a lot to me. I think that's a good measure of our relationship.

Closeness and communication have many different measures. In chapter 5, some of the mothers who wanted to describe how close they are to their daughters—even if they don't discuss intimate sexual details with them—said their daughters know they can always come to them for help if they "get in trouble" (i.e., become pregnant).

The security of having your mother's support when

you have a serious problem is an important aspect of good mother-daughter relationships. How wonderful to know there is someone who is always there for you, no matter what.

I use my mother as a sounding board for things I'm trying to work out in my head. AIDS is so overwhelming that it's good to be able to ask my mother some questions about it, even though she tells me she has a lot of unanswered questions about it herself.

People are a lot more wary about other sexually-transmitted diseases, too, such as herpes. There's an old joke that my friends and I used to tell: Q. What's the difference between love and herpes? A. Herpes is forever.

I feel safe because I don't go to bars and pick up men and sleep with them. I would hope sexual diseases are mostly transmitted through casual encounters. Since I don't have them, I'm not concerned. I don't ask anyone if they have any diseases and neither do my friends.

But I am closely in touch with my conscience and while I try to be flexible about most things, I'm adamant about one thing: I believe in a one-person relationship. I don't know if that comes from a part of my personality that is jealous or possessive or both, but I could not be involved with someone who is unfaithful. I've been that way for a long time. In retrospect, it seems I was right all along.

That's also why I share my mother's deep aversion to adultery—cheating on your husband or wife, having extra-marital sex. I would never want to open up my marriage sexually to include other people. No way!

Adultery is, for me, grounds for ending a marriage.

Knowing my husband slept with other women would deeply hurt me. Nothing could balance it for me. I doubt that it would be worth it to me to remain in the marriage.

If my husband broke his marriage vows to me it would be a deep betrayal and humiliation. To me, sex is something so sacred and important, there is no room for adultery. Adultery merely would underscore the carelessness of the relationship, and I don't want a careless relationship.

I have never slept around. I've always wanted to and even been told by some college friends that I *should*, but I've never been able to do that. I guess it comes down to the fact that trust is the most important thing to me and it takes a while to establish. Commitment might mean I'm with you and you only. That would be enough. Just for right now. Not forever. I'm not ready for anything else right now.

My mother thought she had a lot to deal with when she was growing up. While I would never want to change places with her, growing up in the '50s sounds like a piece of cake to me. When Mom interviewed me and my brothers about the highly-controversial "children's" book, *Show Me*, I blithely responded that children would not be shocked by the book but that probably their parents would be.

Today, there's a lot of advice on how to talk to your parents about sex so that they—your parents—won't blush. Kids are asked to understand that their parents may feel awkward and embarrassed about sex, even though the marital sex they have is legitimized by society. Teenagers are advised to pick the time carefully before asking questions like, "Mom, what kind of birth control do you think I should use?"

My mother sometimes blushes but she's willing to discuss everything with me, sometimes even more than I want to hear. I'm far more conservative about sex than she is and one of the reasons I am is that she has always let me be free to make up my own mind. Many things I'd rather not talk about at all; others, I find my female friends from high school and college are the best people to talk things over with.

Girls today are far more aware of their sexuality—a result of many factors, among them the women's movement, the health and fitness revolution and the increasing numbers of female high school graduates going to college. Today, more women than men are in college. According to the Higher Education Research Institute, 52 percent of those enrolled are women. Women are moving away from traditional fields of teaching, nursing, social work and secretarial and are turning to business, engineering, science, medicine and law.

Going away to college is the first time many young women are on their own. They have a lot of decisions to make. One of the most important is about sex. How will they handle it? Women entering college are increasingly like men in wanting power and money. If you don't start out that way, the amount of money you owe for student loans at the end of four or more years of study probably will bring you to the same philosophical conclusions.

But not in sex. Women college students are far more conservative about sex than are college men. The Higher Education Research Institute also reports that 63 percent of college men believe in pre-marital sex, but only 32 percent of college women do. Those statistics have remained unchanged since 1970, when the question was first researched.

College women today aren't as radical as those in the '60s. We take a lot for granted. My mother reminds me that many schools used to refuse to admit women. Women have always wanted higher education, she says, and now that we have access—what would community colleges, four-year schools and universities do without us?—we're taking advantage of it.

Women students are not lulled to sleep by our many advantages. Today's campus women are not the dedicated activists who created health clinics, rape prevention seminars, rape counseling and campus escort services for women. But we know we have to work to keep these rights. Women students in California state universities have successfully organized to insure continued funding for these protections.

On college campuses today, women have a healthy awareness of date rape and sexual harassment by faculty. Schools are finally instituting sexual harassment policies because their female students insist on it. An estimated one million female college students experience some form of sexual harassment, reports the Project on the Status of Education of Women.

I remember when I told my mother, long distance, about a girl I knew as an undergraduate who dropped a course because the Teacher's Assistant kept hitting on her for a date. And she was getting an A in it on her own! My mother wanted to fly out immediately and confront the T.A. for my friend.

The truth was the girl did not want a confrontation—that's why she dropped the course. She did what was comfortable for her. I gave her my full support and later, when the same T.A. hit on me and another friend, we all filed complaints with the Academic Department. One year later, he was no longer on the faculty. My mother always wants immediate action, justice and a resolution of all problems. Even though I'm studying to be a lawyer, I know that's not always possible. Once again, I guess I'm just more conservative than my Mom—another role reversal.

Women college students are concerned about taking responsibility for their sex lives. Many women depend on their student health centers for gynecological exams, contraceptive information and information on sexually-transmitted diseases. Still, I've not yet heard of a female college student whipping out her medical records—or requesting them from her mate—before making love.

It might be wise for mothers and daughters to check out the student health center when they look at potential colleges. Apparently, it's not enough to ascertain that the administration, faculty and curriculum are what you're looking for when you go to college.

High school girls, too, are concerned about their health. That seems to be to be the appropriate age to begin to be responsible for your body. Yet, it is really sad, I think, that in Philadelphia, hundreds of teenagers are turning up at health clinics with a penicillin-resistant strain of gonorrhea that has climbed to epidemic proportions. A doctor at Temple University Hospital said, "We see hundreds of teens with VD every year."

What a way to start out your sex life. The kids, the doctors say, seem to have a "blind trust" in their partners and don't understand the consequences of having sex. Fortunately, the disease is cured with only one injection. But I wonder, do the kids learn a lesson from this? Do they tell their partners to get treatment? Do they know how to protect themselves from future infection? A high school student has to be quite mature to answer yes. I wonder if I could have handled all these responsibilities when I was a teenager.

My mother never told me about venereal diseases, except never to sit on public toilets. I don't think she knew much about VD or considered it very important. That's another thing that's changed today.

She never mentioned sexually-transmitted diseases, either, and probably for the same reasons. I think I told her about them first. Everyone talked and joked about herpes when I was an undergraduate, but I don't know anyone who has it. The closest "contact" I've had with herpes was as an undergraduate. A guy who was a waiter told me he thought he might have herpes. I remember thinking, "And he's serving food!" It made me paranoid about eating in that restaurant for a little while. I was freaked out because I knew so little about how herpes is transmitted.

Doctors say that AIDS is not transmitted through casual contact, but some people think you can get sexually-transmitted diseases anywhere. A commitment to research and education should help clear up misconceptions.

I hear that herpes is not a disease you can catch easily. Still, I'm suspicious of most medical pronouncements on what's safe and what isn't. First doctors said you can transmit herpes only when it is active. Now they say you can transmit it even when it is in remission. Each year, the medical world discovers that you *can* catch things they said previously were not contagious. Most of these diseases cannot be spread through casual contact, but all I knew was I wanted to be as far away from that waiter as possible.

I was incredibly naive as an undergraduate and so were most of my friends. We dismissed venereal or sexually-transmitted diseases as being the result of not being clean. We considered ourselves clean and too above it all ever to get involved with someone who would have VD. We believed we knew by instinct what to look for: If a guy looked clean, he was clean. Remember the expression clean cut? You don't hear it so much today.

This superior attitude was our way of not dealing with a serious problem. I didn't go through college worried every moment about sexual diseases. It was the kind of thing, I thought, that only happened to other people.

My innocence extended in those days to homosexuality, too. I've certainly grown up aware of a homosexual and bisexual society, as well as an actively heterosexual one. I think this is especially true of California, where I go to school. I've been made aware of the prevalence of gay men and lesbians. At first, the fact that people around me had different sexual preferences from mine made me uncomfortable.

I was first made aware of homosexuality by a female undergraduate. I was friends with her and finally realized she was gay. It was startling at first but I realized I didn't want to let it affect our friendship. Today, I try not to judge people for their sexual orientation. People can do whatever they want. I just prefer they not do it around me.

I can't deny that sometimes I'm uncomfortable around lesbians. I can't change that. As much as I try to to be, I get uncomfortable. Male homosexuality is much easier for me to handle because it doesn't threaten me individually. But I don't think I want to get involved with any guy who admits he's gay or even bisexual. Since I don't like "sharing," it also applies if the "other person" is male. I've never had any sexually-transmitted disease and that seems a good way to prevent getting one.

I'm a little wary of people who are attracted to both sexes. I am not attracted to the same sex, so I find it hard to understand. I've learned a lot about myself and won't call my feelings prejudices, but I'd like to be more comfortable with people with different sexual orientations from mine. Sometimes, it's a real effort.

Despite my feelings, I believe in rights for all people, whatever their sexual orientation. I do not believe any sanctions or limitations should be imposed on homosexuals. Neither do I think anyone should be discriminated against because of sexual orientation in terms of hiring, housing, living, employment or service in the military.

Homosexuals can do what they want sexually—but over there, away from me. My mother thinks that sounds terrible and as I say it, so do I, but that's how I feel.

Gay liberation has made me aware that there is a great deal of discrimination against homosexuals. It has also had another affect on me: I'm far more wary about whom I get involved with. The prevalence of homosexuality and bisexuality have made me even more hesitant than I was previously about relationships.

In the civil rights movement, many blacks said, "Whites don't have to like us. Just get off our backs." I apply that advice to my reaction to homosexuals, at the same time affirming their constitutional rights. What it comes down to is it's okay with me whatever anyone does sexually—as long as they are consenting adults. There are some things, however, that I would rather not hear explicitly described.

It's normal to have reservations about things you don't fully understand. I have to be honest about my reactions to homosexuality, so I can deal with them.

Without the sexual revolution of two decades ago, I'd never be discussing these matters today. The revolution was important because it let women become less inhibited, freer to recognize they too, may want a sex life. I'm glad women have choices today, but the woman is still the one who gets pregnant. We can't change that, even if the guy is more supportive and even if there is less stigma than previously.

To me, sex comes with love, not vice versa. I think sleeping around is self-destructive. Starting out with sex is not the way to begin a relationship. The Double Standard still exists: Guys don't respect girls who sleep with them right away.

Some day, I want to get married—but only once. Many of my friends, whose parents are divorced, feel the same way. I won't just sit back and let my marriage take its

course, either. I'm willing to do what I can to keep it working. My mother tells me that's what it takes.

OUR BODIES, OUR VERY SELVES

MOTHER | I want my daughter to know about birth control so she can be in charge of her own biology, rather than vice versa. Margaret Sanger, a champion of legalized birth control, repeatedly stresses that if women cannot control the number of children we have and when we have them—we cannot control our lives. We cannot begin to plan our personal lives or professional careers. For women, birth control is one of the cornerstones of equality in a world where anatomy—particularly female anatomy—has often meant destiny not of our own choosing.

Germaine Greer's reply to the querulous question, "Why are there so few great women artists?" is that they died in childbirth or had so many children they had no time to develop their talent. That applies to all women, not just artists.

Today, the death rate from giving birth is low, despite the popularity among U.S. doctors of performing convenient (for them) and expensive (for us) Cesareans, which are far more dangerous to women's lives than natural childbirth.

Nonetheless, the number of children we have is no longer only a matter of our physical well-being. The matter is also emotional, and what's at stake is the quality of our lives.

I say these things in retrospect. Only recently have I managed to figure out the impact of my biology on my life. The fact that today women have some options—none as fail-safe as I would hope for, though—makes possible our struggle for liberation. It's the spur, the root of our insistence for equal rights and equal opportunity.

It's no coincidence that the current women's movement in the United States followed the advent of the birth control pill, which is 98 percent effective in preventing pregnancies. The famous Pill, which also helped fuel the sexual revolution, is still the most popular form of birth control despite the now-proven fact it is dangerous for many women. Betty Friedan might disagree, but it was the Pill that first changed our lives. The women's movement came next.

Birth control is still a risky science—for women. I for one am waiting for the perfect device or potion that gives 100 percent protection and has no side effects on women. Of course, that means it will have to be a device for men.

Growing up in a vacuum of ignorance, I never heard of birth control. I did know I was lucky to be born, not only because of the adverse economic effects on my family of the Depression, but also because my mother—who told me so little—talked occasionally about the fact if she had not had a miscarriage before I was born, I would not be born. They only wanted three children, she said.

I was the youngest of three daughters. The miscarriage, she told me, had been a boy. She said "boy" with awe—surely a noun commanding respect in our house of all female children. Thus, I got the message when I was only five years old that my presence here on earth was somewhat hit or miss. That gave me plenty to think about, but since I didn't know how babies were made in the first place, I did not think to ask how they were prevented. I wonder what my parents did to limit their family. I still don't know.

The first form of birth control I learned about, once again thanks to my friend Jack, was condoms, which—despite their lack of aesthetics—are now enjoying a new and deserved respect for preventing the transmission of sexual diseases, preventing conception and not being life-threatening to the wearer as the Pill and IUDs are to their users.

Later, my girlfriends from high school, still claiming to be virgins, told me self-righteously that if a boy really loves you, he will use a condom if you have sex. But of course, we were not supposed to have sex. If somehow we slipped up and fell asleep while he "took advantage" of us, it was hoped he'd be considerate enough to use a condom.

We believed women had to be passive in the matter of contraception. In order to "get" us to sleep with them, boys had to talk us into it. We were romantics. How could we be so crude and obvious as to be prepared for sex? Only *loose* women planned or expected to have intercourse.

Good girls like us, who through some mistake, preferably being overwhelmed by uncontrollable passion or sleep, might accidentally have sex, could not take preventive measures. The unrealistic and double-standard scenario written for us did not include being smart or equal partners. We could not be, without admitting that we, too, had sexual desires. Birth control was much too delicate and embarrassing to discuss with strangers, friends—or lovers. That put women in the '50s at the mercy of men, a fact that is still true to some extent today.

I've often told Cathy how women of my generation—when abortions were illegal and dangerous—lived in fear of getting pregnant. She is shocked that I was so helpless, but I was. We all were. Intellectually, our sexuality was repressed—but very little quieted our glands. Sex, in abstention, became the frustrating focus of our lives rather than a satisfying part of it. Having lived through this distortion makes me today a strong advocate of birth control.

It's hard for today's young women to understand that as recently as thirty years ago, the birth control method of choice was still abstinence—many years after Thomas Malthus preached his parochial solution of "moral restraint" to families overburdened with children.

In the '60s, there was no restraint—the sexual revolution had hit. But we still didn't know much about birth control. In that decade, I had two diaphragm babies out of three. I learned through experience that diaphragms, which I'd heard whispered in college were almost as safe as condoms and surely more fun, are only 80 percent effective for the average woman.

Today, I also know diaphragms have no "dangerous" side effects, except, of course, in my case—babies.

After having three children within four years, I asked my gynecologist-obstetrician about the best method of birth control. He replied that he was Catholic, which I knew, and only wanted to facilitate birth, not prevent it.

I was disappointed by his answer. During my pregnancies, he answered all my questions in a straightforward manner and made me feel as if we were a team. His rejection hurt.

I was hurt because of all we had been through together. I used to laughingly refer to him as "the father of my children" because we started out together: I was among his first patients and the first to have natural childbirth. We learned together. I chose him carefully when I came to Chicago from Philadelphia and was pregnant with Cathy, my first child. He was the only doctor who would discuss natural childbirth or nursing. Others fended me off with remarks such as, "Oh, my wife never worried about that."

Before becoming his patient, I asked if there were a complication, would he save me or the baby. He replied, "Both." He found natural childbirth classes for me to attend—they were rare then—and sneaked my husband in the delivery room, even though it was illegal at the time.

When he wouldn't talk to me about birth control, I felt

abandoned but respected his choice. I needed, however, to assert mine. I asked our family doctor—we had one in those days—for the Pill.

"Oh, no," he said. "It's still in the experimental stage. It hasn't been tested thoroughly. I cannot prescribe it."

That did not deter me. Over the years, I had become friendly with him and his family and I learned from his wife that she was taking the Pill to "clear up acne on her back." Armed with this information, I triumphantly reported to the doctor that I knew his wife took the Pill and I wanted it, too.

"It'll give you headaches," he warned me.

"Children give me headaches," I flippantly replied.

Reluctantly, he gave me the prescription. Ten years later, when Barbara Seaman exposed the Pill's dangers, he told me, "See, I was right all along."

I would hate my daughter to have to play these games today. The majority of American women do not use birth control during their first sexual encounter but most often opt for the Pill and then sterilization after that, a study shows. In 1986, some thirty million women were using some form of birth control.

I still have no idea what to tell my daughter is the best and safest form of birth control. Everything that is effective has dangerous side effects. The Pill, IUDs, even spermicides have proved to cause problems. The latter, while not yet proven dangerous to users, may be a cause of birth defects—and a successful lawsuit against its manufacturer for that reason may also dissipate the use of gels, foams, suppositories and sponges.

We always hear about breakthroughs in contraception. The newest is a device that uses saliva to predict ovulation. The method, which is being tested, is promoted as being as easy to use as a lollipop, avoids religious and cultural edicts that frown on birth control and can predict ovulation five days in advance. It is, of course, for women.

Today, women have many options for birth control, yet few really viable choices. Though I believe the best and safest birth control for women is one used by men, it seems women today are pretty much where I was in the '50s. Except now the problem of birth control is complicated by the fear of AIDS and other sexually-transmitted diseases. Reverting to the use of condoms is a good idea—especially if women can buy them and suggest their use as freely as men can. Condoms, which used to be the subject of many jokes, are now seriously viewed as a panacea, one which may not only prevent unwanted lives, but also save wanted ones.

Birth control should be taught in a forthright manner to teenagers, whose unplanned pregnancies are becoming epidemic. It is time to cast off our Puritanical and Victorian morality and judgments and educate teens so that children will choose not to have children. (See chapter 7.)

Despite the fact that many things have not changed, American women have made a dramatic gain: The right of choice, of having a safe, legal abortion. Unfortunately, poor women have lost their right to have federally-reimbursed abortions, a punitive ruling that violates not only women's rights but also the separation of church and state.

The challenge is to keep abortions legal, for women to

control our own bodies. Even if abortions are illegal, women—poor and rich alike—will still have them, but we can't regress to back-alley and self-induced abortions with their high mortality rates. Women who are victims of rape and incest need the safe, legal option of abortion. We must not abandon them.

The Alan Guttmacher Institute estimates that some forty to sixty million abortions are performed worldwide each year. Of that number, thirty-three million are legal. More than half of the world's population live in countries where abortion on demand is legal. Some 25 percent live in countries where terminating a pregnancy is allowed only to protect the mother's health. Not surprisingly, countries where abortions are rare are those governed by Islamic fundamentalists.

Worldwide, there are thirty-seven to fifty-five abortions for every one thousand women of childbearing age. In the United States, the rate is 27 percent, the highest of Western industrialized countries.

Scientists soon may be indirectly responsible for ending bombings and attacks on women's health centers—a responsibility generally ignored by federal and state law enforcement agencies. The cease-fire may come about with the use of a drug that appears to be highly effective and safe for aborting unwanted pregnancies. The medicine, known generically as RU486, bypasses surgical abortions —the focus of anti-choice groups. These groups will have to battle pharmaceutical companies to prevent the drug's manufacture and distribution, rather than unsuspecting pregnant women.

Meanwhile, we must guard with our lives our right of choice.

DAUGHTER | My mother and I haven't discussed birth control much, but she has always warned me about the dangers of the Pill—dangers she knew nothing about when she took it for so many years.

Scientists still haven't come up with anything very effective—a birth control method that is 100 percent effective and is not dangerous to use.

Both partners should take responsibility for precautionary methods. Just the woman worrying about it is not enough—although she *is* the one who gets pregnant. I think mothers should emphasize to their daughters that if they're going to have a relationship, they must protect themselves. And their partners should be involved in how to do that.

To avoid dangerous devices or drugs, many of my friends used the sponge when it first became popular but now problems with it have been noted. I cannot recommend a form of birth control, but the sponge seems to be the most convenient and accessible. It does not, however, give protection against AIDS. Other women I know like the cervical cap, but it's not easily available.

Spermicides have also been added to the list of dangerous methods of birth control. I believe that if men could become pregnant, we would have a variety of perfectly safe and effective birth control devices to choose from.

As we mentioned in chapter 7, preventing unwanted pregnancy is not the only problem with sex. Concern about AIDS has made many young women re-evaluate the condom as their contraceptive of choice. As the ad for Mentor Contraceptives says, "Let's face it, sex these days can be risky business and you need all the protection you can get. Between the fear of unplanned pregnancy, sexually transmitted diseases and the potential side effects of many female contraceptives, it may seem like sex is hardly worth the risk anymore."

In suggesting their product as the solution to these problems, the ad concludes: "So why take your fears to bed?"

The ad is smart marketing. It suggests a viable option and stresses that condoms offer a "water-tight barrier which prevents the transmission of bodily fluids . . ." It asks women to buy birth control devices for men to use. It talked about pleasure, too, and quotes a respondent to an independent study who says the Mentor condom "feels almost as good as nothing at all." It's the answer to the joke that circulated around my freshman dormitory: Wearing a condom while making love is like wearing a raincoat in the shower.

Fear over AIDS is rampant among both sexes on college campuses. Smart sex may be the only kind we dare have. Women will have to get over their inhibitions about buying condoms and about suggesting that men use them. Aggressive marketing by condom manufacturers is helping women overcome this reluctance. But I see this new trend as a step forward for women, especially those who don't want to catch a sexually-transmitted disease. And, it certainly puts the sexual act on a fifty-fifty basis.

While it's confusing to sort out the available means of birth control to identify the safest and most effective one, I am not the least confused about abortion. It is *not* birth control. But it is control over your own life. My mother and I have talked about this often, and we agree that abortion is an *option* women must have. To take that option away seems to me to be an outrageous deprivation of a fundamental right. A woman must have the right to choose between terminating her pregnancy or having a child. To deprive her of this choice is to mandate the course of her life.

I understand some of the opponents of abortion and their objections. I do not understand those who verbally attack women who seek abortions or those people who bomb women's health centers. You have to deal with reality. The reality is that young girls do get sexually involved with boys and women with men. Sometimes they get pregnant when they don't want to. It happens all the time.

My generation's attitude, I hope, reflects my own: Abortion is not to be relied on as a form of birth control; it is never something you want. You don't desire it. You prefer not to be pregnant in the first place. But when you need it, it must be available.

If abortions were illegal, as they were before 1973, it would change women's lives in a negative way. I believe if it were illegal it would certainly defeat the purpose of saving potential lives. It would destroy so many actual ones.

I know more than a handful of people whose lives

would have been ruined without this option. Their hopes, dreams and futures would have been destroyed. People can make mistakes and they should not be made to pay forever for them. To outlaw abortion is to deprive women of the right of choice. I don't know what it was like when abortion was illegal.

If abortions were illegal, butcher abortions would return. A "black market" for the procedure would exist, and this market, completely devoid of regulations concerning health and safety, would probably seriously endanger a woman's health, future child-bearing potential —even her life.

My friends and I can be as conservative as we want about politics and economics, but because we are women, we can't be conservative about the right to choose between having a baby or terminating a pregnancy. So many young women have been faced with this dilemma: "Oh, my God, my period's a week late!" I think I have heard this exclamation a thousand times. Usually, it's a false alarm. But when it's not, a woman's right to choose what to do must be preserved.

Boys today are far more responsible toward their sexual partners. Depending on their level of involvement, they usually are supportive if a girl becomes pregnant, offering to pay for the abortion, to be there when she gets it, to help in whatever way they can.

Still, women are the ones at risk, both emotionally and physically. I know of a young woman who became pregnant while in high school. She had been very "casually" involved with the guy. So, she never told him. She had an abortion and never told him. I can't get over that.

I was friends with another young woman who was deeply involved with a guy. She had just returned to college after summer vacation and he was far away back home. When she told him she was pregnant, he was very upset that he wasn't with her. He wanted to fly out right away to give her support and to pay for the abortion.

She was only eighteen and hysterical about being pregnant, but she wanted to be alone in her hysteria. She would not let him be with her. I couldn't understand that, but I do respect a woman's right to do whatever she wants. Men should not make the decisions in these cases. She did let her boyfriend pay.

A female friend went with her when she got the abortion. She was very vulnerable at that stage of life and came back a wreck. I tried to talk to her a lot. It took her a long time to adjust. Not too long afterwards, she got pregnant again. She hadn't been using birth control. I hate to say this but I was disgusted with her and scared: She wasn't sure who the father was and she didn't take precautions. Neither did he. She had another abortion. I don't know who paid for the second one.

I didn't approve of what she was doing. She was obviously sleeping around and I thought that was a serious mistake. She was just starting college. She had four more years to go. After the second abortion, I think she learned an important lesson because she was much more careful.

Despite my harsh judgments, I was grateful that she had some options. Her life would have been ruined without the right to abortion. She told me she did not see abortion as an automatic birth control device but as a desperate saving grace. It preserved her life and her future. Without the right to abortion, you're damaging a real life to preserve the potential for what may turn out to be a life.

I reply to objections to abortion on the grounds that it is murder with an analogy:

Say you have blueprints of a home you plan to construct on a new piece of property. Shrubbery, landscaping and oak trees are drawn in. Gardeners have already planted acorns around your new home. Perhaps you then want to give a housewarming picnic and decide a nice spot to hold it would be under the shade of the oak tree on your new property. You invite everyone to picnic under an oak tree, but when they get there, of course, there is no oak tree. You can't call an acorn an oak tree. It is true it has the potential to be a tree, but at that moment it is not. The two cannot logically be equated.

There will be oak trees, perhaps, some day, if the acorns planted there mature. But that's hypothetical. I believe it's more important for a woman to have control over her present life than to make her sacrifice it for a potential one.

A recent Harris poll shows that 74 percent of those surveyed believe abortion should continue to be legal. Abortion is widely used and widely accepted by American women, from every walk of life.

My mother has her own radio show and once, when I was on semester break from school, she invited me to sit in on a live interview she was doing with Patti Davis, whose parents are Nancy and Ronald Reagan. Patti had just written a book called *Homefront*. In it she talks about abortion, so my mother asked her what her views are on it. They are in direct opposition to those of her father, who has a strong anti-choice stance.

Patti said that women who want abortions will get them, including poor women. "Don't forget what it was like when abortions were illegal," she said on the air. "Don't forget the butchers and back-alley abortions. We must never go back to those days."

Cheryl Rodriguez-Jensen, president of the Du Page County, Illinois, National Organization for Women, wrote a moving letter to the editor of the *Chicago Tribune*. In it, she says that ". . . a small number of self-righteous religious fanatics have taken it upon themselves to determine that women will have no reproductive choices . . . Despite violent threats from those who claim to know God personally, despite the efforts of those who want us to forget that a woman's life is a human life, women will not go back . . ."

Condemning the violence and terrorism of "pro-life bombers," she further declares: "We will not go back to dark, frightening alleys, we will not go back to murderous, unskilled opportunists . . . women will continue to fight for the right to safe, legal abortions."

I do not know what it was like in those days, or what it must have been like to be so circumscribed in dealing with your own body, but it sounds oppressive. My mother and her friends speak of the days before 1973 with emotions akin to horror. It is clear to me that not having choices or options was a terrible burden for women and the weight of that burden controlled their lives physically, emotionally and psychologically.

I am a feminist who is fairly conservative in many matters, but the one issue that would get me into the streets would be the attempt to take away the choice to have an abortion. I see that not only as a feminist issue, but a constitutional issue—an attempt to strip away the privacy and autonomy of the individual.

I can only reiterate how I feel on this emotionally-charged subject: Women must have a fundamental right of choice between terminating or continuing their pregnancy.

If abortion is declared illegal, a dangerous black market will exist. Women don't *want* abortions. They *need* the right to choose.

I'm lucky that my mother has been so open with me in discussing this subject because it puts me on guard that my rights may be infringed. In the United States, today, parents and children are talking frankly about the right to abortion because its legality hangs on the fragile strings of an increasingly conservative U.S. Supreme Court. Many women are concerned the decision will be overturned, and there is now talk of a Constitutional amendment, introduced by Representative Patricia Schroeder (D.-Col.), to protect our right to choose.

Mothers and daughters together make a powerful force. It is up to us to insure this right not only for ourselves, but for future generations of mothers and daughters.

CHILDREN

MOTHER | I talk often to my daughter about the responsibilities and pleasures of sex and good relationships, but there is also another aspect of having sexual intercourse: Children. They are the wondrous biological result of human coupling.

Not all women want children. Those who do and are able to do so know that parenthood brings many joys and many heartaches, too. I jokingly say that childbirth, the experience of labor, is an appropriate introduction to childrearing. Cathy knows that I mean that labor is well-named. Its hard work and emotional highs and lows are precursors of what is to come in raising a child.

My daughter wants to have children. If she did not choose to, I would understand her decision. I have taught her to be free and the basic ingredient of freedom is choice. But since that is her desire, at least right now, it frees me to wax eloquent to her about what it means to me to have three wonderful children.

I feel lucky to have raised Cathy, although I know full well in many ways she has raised me. I tell her I would like to be like her when I grow up. By that I mean I admire her loyalty to her friends, her certainty about what is right and wrong for her, her sheer determination to accomplish her goals and her complete honesty. She is so much her own person, not swayed or swept away by anyone else's beliefs—including mine! It has taken me a lifetime to get to where she is at the start, and I admire her for that.

I have never thought much about being a grandparent, but I probably will be one day because all three of my children say they want to have children. They never say they have a preference when it comes to gender, but if Cathy does have a daughter, she will then learn from the other end about the special biological connection between mothers and daughters.

I recall with amusement and tenderness the message left on my answering machine when a friend of mine had her first grandchild. "I'm a grandmother," she proudly announced, "and it's a baby woman!" Borrowing a line from the *Doonesbury* cartoon strip, she was trying to avoid sexist stereotyping but was also making a strong, biologically-correct statement: The girl child is mother to the woman.

Today, our daughters have to figure out well in advance how to have careers and families. Sociologists say that women spend ten years in rearing children. To me, it seems more like 150 years. Cathy's generation is the one that will have to make changes in the workplace, so that women don't have to choose between professions and family, a choice men rarely have to make. Businesses are going to have to bend and there are a few signs they are beginning to.

When is the best time to have a baby? That question is asked so frequently today. I hear it all the time in my professional capacity as a writer about women's issues. I wish I had the answers. Combining a career and family is such hard work that an increasing number of women are opting not to have children at all. Many are waiting until their careers are established; they are aware that those early post-college years are the ones in which men surge ahead to the top and stay there.

I'm proud to be Cathy's mother. I've always been proud of her. My friends tell me, "You always took Cathy everywhere with you. You were always together." I took her to assignments, marches, speeches, radio and television shows. I wanted to expose her to all I could, but there was another factor at work: I loved being with her. I still do.

It is because I am so close with my daughter that we can speak of sex. We are not close because we discuss it. That did not come first. The closeness did. From infancy on, I tried to make Cathy feel comfortable about sex, through my actions and words. Today, our conversations about sex are not so much fact-finding—except for our talks about AIDS—as they are philosophical. I have strong opinions. She has strong emerging ones. We do not always agree.

Mothers teach daughters until daughters are old enough to teach mothers. An echo of my hopes for my daughter—for all our daughters—is in *The Third Sex: The New Professional Woman*, by Patricia A. McBroom. She says: "We need to value what our bodies can do and trust our intellect . . . Men project their sexuality upon the world . . . Women can do no less. If we are to be equal, we must love our bodies in feminine form—the miraculous source of life—and project that love onto the world, knowing that its expression is true . . ."

The joy of having children is to see them define their personhoods and mold their own personalities. Cathy has not changed much in her very being since she was six years old; she has merely improved on it. She is her own, inviolate self. It is my joy to watch her weave her womanhood.

I look at Cathy's emergence in my life as a close and trusted friend as miraculous. I surely did not expect things to go so well with me and my daughter—or my sons— when I was left to raise them alone. The stigma of being a single parent was strong in the '70s.

One summer day, my son Robert, then five years old, took me by the hand and asked me to go outside with him.[*] Holding on tightly, he carefully walked around the house with me, looking at doors and windows and shaking his head. There was something he didn't understand.

"Mommy," he finally asked, pressing my hand with his

---

[*]This story first appeared in *Ms.* magazine, November, 1984.

warm, chubby fingers, "is our home broken?"

His words shot through my body, alerting every protective instinct, activating my private defense system, the one I hold in reserve to ward off attacks against my children.

"Oh, Robbie," I answered him, hugging him tightly, "did someone tell you that we have a broken home?"

"Yes," he said sweetly. "But it doesn't look broken!"

"It's not," I assured him. "Our house is not broken and neither are we."

I explained that "broken" is some people's way of describing a home with only one parent, usually the mother. Sometimes there is only one parent because of divorce, like us. "There are lots of homes like ours. And they're still homes."

Robbie looked relieved and went to play with his friends. I stood there, shaking with anger.

What a way to put down a little kid and me, too, I thought. I wondered how often Cathy and Ray had heard those words. I supported my three children, fed and clothed them. I was there for them emotionally and physically. I managed to keep up payments on the house. Although we struggled financially, we were happy and loving. What was "broken" about us?

That was in 1970. The expression is as prevalent today as it was then. We've made some headway in raising the issue of sexist expressions, including such formerly popular ones as calling women "girls," "gals" or "broads." We've even sensitized a few headline writers to their unhealthy habit of describing women as "grandmothers" and "mothers" when the stories about them are unrelated to their biological roles.

But a household headed by a woman is still a "broken home," despite the fact that more than eight million women raise their families alone. A residence in which a man is not in residence, the phrase implies, is not a home. The phrase is often used as an explanation for a terrible crime, as if a woman alone is disreputable and can only raise a vicious miscreant who will naturally prey upon society: "The alleged murdered is a loner and comes from a broken home."

Over the years, similar buzzwords have sent me buzzing. Even though I work for a newspaper and understand how journalists are misunderstood, I am constantly writing letters of protest to publications that deprecate me and all women with frequent use of expressions such as "divorcee," "unwed" mother and "illegitimate" children. They have something offensively in common: They tell us if no husband/father exists, neither do women and children.

Society does not help single or divorced women raise their children or keep their families intact. The scorn felt for so-called "broken" homes is expressed in the lack of support systems for heads of those households, in the withholding of federally funded quality childcare, job training and equal pay, and in the meanness with which aid to dependent children is doled out.

The expression "broken home" suggests that my children never had a chance in life because their father was not present and what I did doesn't count. I know that's not true, and it's not true for millions of other women also stigmatized by the term.

I have some testimony that I am not alone in my strong belief that my house is truly a home. It comes from my three children, Catharine, Raymond Jr., and Robert. On a recent Thanksgiving, my trio gathered in Chicago for the holiday. After they left, I found a note on my desk. Cathy had written it and she and her brothers signed it before dispersing to their various colleges coast to coast.

"Dear Mom," the letter begins, "Yet another Thanksgiving holiday has drawn our family together for a few meaningful days. It's just enough time to touch base, strengthen our bond and reaffirm how important we are to one another.

"It is you who draws us here year after year. Whether you are aware of it or not, you have an enormous power which reaches out and pulls us toward you. This power is the love, devotion, blind faith and unswerving loyalty you have showered upon us our whole lives long.

"It is not something we will ever be without, or forget.

"It is something that is now a part of us; thus, we carry a part of you forever.

"We thank you for making us what we are."

As I read Cathy's moving words, I remembered Robbie's question a dozen years ago and how much it hurt me. Here was the real answer to the question: "Is our home broken?"

My daughter wants to get married and raise her children in a two-parent home. I hope that works out for her. My daughter and I speak of sex. We speak of everything. I hope she does that with her children, too, because love is built on trust and communication.

Cathy, I wish you happiness in your marriage, should you marry, with your children, should you have them, and in your life. I hope you are as lucky as I am and have a daughter, too—just like you.

DAUGHTER | I can't wait to have children. If I have a daughter, I can only hope I will give her the comfort, security and space she needs to develop into her own person, intellectually, emotionally and sexually. I want her to know she can come to me when she has questions about sex, to give her answers and feedback and support—the way I know I can go to my mother.

I think my approach will be matter-of-fact. This seems to work best. I wouldn't want to highlight or downplay sex or personal relationships. I don't want to distort their importance or take them out of context. I would just deal with them as straight facts.

My major goal is to be supportive without being suffocating. After all, a mother-daughter relationship is between two people—it's not a one-way street.

I realize how difficult it is to talk about sex with your daughter. Even my liberated mom has trouble at times. I hope my daughter respects me enough so that she will listen when I tell her how I feel. I hope I respect her enough not to be upset if she doesn't agree with everything I say. I want her to be confident enough in our relationship to question and challenge me on everything.

Intimacy is the key, and it's built on love and trust. I want to be very close to my daughter, but I also want her to retain her independence. At the same time, I, as a responsible adult, want to guide her through the labyrinth of human sexuality. That, I suppose, constitutes a conflict of interests!

I hope my strong urge to "guide" never turns out to be excessive or moralistic, traits that shut down communication. I have seen the harm that comes from over-protective parents and I want to avoid it, as my mother has strived to do.

I would tell my daughter about sex in the same way I would tell my sons. I would try to ease it into her existence, as part of a total picture. The most important thing is to let her know I am there to talk about anything. I hope that my daughter will hear me; it will be up to me to figure out when she is ready to hear me and *what* she is ready to hear.

One of the things that frustrates mothers most, I've observed, is when they open up to their daughters, answer all questions, spill their guts and are non-judgmental—in other words, do everything right—and their daughters don't listen. It's upsetting. I can tell. But if my daughter were not ready to listen or didn't want to hear me, I'd either let it alone or try some other way to get through to her.

If she didn't want to hear what I had to say about menstruation, for instance, I'd get her a good book on the subject or a video cassette. Or, maybe, I'd ask somebody else to talk to her about it if I thought it was urgent, maybe a pediatrician or a close female relative.

While we do not have perfect control over our reproductive lives, women can still pretty much plan when to have children. That's an important option and is bound to affect in a positive way the relationship between mothers and daughters. I want to have children very much, but only after I've established myself professionally, when I'm at a place in the world where I feel good about what I'm doing, and when I'm enough in love with someone that I want to have children with him.

That's the only way I want to have children: With the father participating as a full partner in childraising. One of my single girlfriends talks about having a baby by herself. There is no one she wants to marry but she does want to have children. She doesn't think she should be deprived of such a great pleasure in life merely because she has not found the "right" guy, someone she wants to spend the rest of her life with and who will be a good husband and father.

If that's what she wants to do, it's fine with me. I believe, though, many complications might arise, because someone, somewhere *is* the father, and what do you do about that? If a woman doesn't want to adopt and prefers to raise a child alone—millions of women end up doing that anyway—I support her decision and hope it works.

But it wouldn't work for me. I do not see having a baby as an independent act. I want to have a child *with* somebody, as an expression of our love. Somebody caring.

Of course, when I do have children, that will make my mother a grandmother. Some of her friends urge their daughters to have a baby—for them! I suppose their pleas are an honest communication of an emotional need to see what the next generation looks like and to love and adore an infant again, but I'm grateful that my mother has never uttered those words even once. I think it puts an unnecessary burden on a daughter, and, if she is single, can be translated into a not-so-subtle plea to get married.

It can also be interpreted as an accusation of failure, of letting down her mother and imperiling the family's biological future. And that's not fair. Even their mothers' promises of eternal gratitude and unlimited, free baby-sitting should not sway daughters to have children unless they want to! I also think that if a daughter tells her mother, "Okay, you want a grandchild so much, I'm going to have a baby, but I do not intend to get married," she may find that the enthusiasm of the would-be grandmom is somewhat dampened.

I read an article recently that talked about the number of young grandmothers in the United States today, a result of the enormous—and growing—numbers of teenage mothers. In 1985, there were 513,000 babies born to teenage mothers. My mother missed being a "young" grandmother, but she still has plenty of time—and plenty of children to have children.

Just as there are more young grandmothers, there are also more older grandmothers. The trend among my female contemporaries is to focus first on our education, get our careers established—and then think about getting married. And, after that, having babies. If, when I finally do have children, my mother has serious adjustments to make—I know I will—because she is an "older" grandmother, I will be there to help her over the hurdle, just as I know she will help me over mine.

In writing this book with my mother, I understood for the first time that I have had excellent sex education all my life. This makes me very serious and concerned about doing the same for my daughter. Being faced with the reality of helping shape the sexual attitudes of an innocent young mind is much harder, I know, than theorizing about what I would say, or do, but still I think about what I want my daughter to know.

I want my daughter to know that when I was growing up, I felt good about my body and my sexuality and I hope she feels the same. I would like not to make too big a deal out of sex or overwhelm her with information, but I do want to communicate to her what's going on in the world around her and with her own body. I'm certain most mothers have that ideal.

I'd tell her more than the basics, I'd tell her some of the hard stuff, too: I'd tell her about birth control and impress upon her that it is a definite biological reality that she could get pregnant. That is a fact of her life. I wouldn't recommend any specific birth control method on the market today because I have no definite answers, even for myself. I wouldn't know what to tell her to use. However, I would alert her to the situation and the need for concern. Perhaps, by the time I have children, there will be easily available, reliable and safe contraceptive methods.

I'll tell my daughter about Stranger Danger, child abuse, molestation and rape, as hard as it will be to do so.

Like every mother, I'll want my child to be safe, within my definition of the word, which is healthy, happy, enjoying her life—and also aware of its dangers. I know I'll have to be very careful bringing up these subjects because I won't want to frighten her unnecessarily. But some things I consider necessary.

I'd talk to her about sexually-transmitted diseases, too. I'd tell her exactly how I feel about them and their physical and moral implications. I can only advise her within the framework of my own standards, the ones I apply to myself. I'll tell her I feel strongly about sexually-transmitted diseases and the lack of commitment and dishonesty they imply.

The best protection against those diseases, I'll tell her, is being very careful about your choice of partner and *knowing* the person you have sex with.

I hope, by that time, there'll be a preventive shot or cure for sexually-transmitted diseases. In the meantime, I believe the threat of disease will lessen the frequency of casual sex, which, I will tell her, is fine with me.

I do not visualize sitting my daughter down one day and laying the whole trip on her. Our relationship will evolve slowly and so will our speaking of sex. My mother helped me to be strong first and believe in myself, so I am not afraid to face facts, even ones I don't like. She used to tell me when I was little, "You ARE Somebody." I came to believe it. I want to do the same for my daughter.

My mother used to intersperse her discussions of the facts of life with another subject important to her, the quality of life. She used to tell me that my life would be different—and better—because of the aesthetics of our home: teak, rosewood and walnut furniture; bright orange accents; pictures and paintings everywhere.

"Smell these, Cathy," she would say of the fresh flowers we always have in the house. "It'll change your life."

And they have shaped my life. My mother has shaped my life—and I've shaped hers. I have much of her independence, but not all, yet sometimes I catch her in Victorian lapses, too. When I was eleven, she and my brother, Ray, were in a head-on auto collision. Neither was hurt, but Mom was really shook up when she came home. I was shook up to see her so shook up! The worst part was she had to leave almost immediately to give a talk to hundreds of people.

"Come with me to my talk," she invited me. "You can be my nurse."

"Why 'nurse,' don't you mean 'doctor'?" I asked her. We both laughed and both felt much better after that.

Her frankness with me all of my life has set me free, but it has also nurtured within me a strong sense of family. When the three of us were very little, we all came down with some kind of infection. I didn't mind because it allowed me to stay home from school and play with our cat, Freedom, a stray a friend had found in the woods near her home.

My mother took us to the pediatrician. He looked at us and without asking a question said, "Get rid of the cat!"

"How did you know we have a cat?" my mother asked.

"I can tell by looking," he answered sternly. "I will not treat patients who have cats. They carry diseases. Get rid of the cat."

"Oh, no, Mother," I begged. "Don't get rid of the cat. He's an orphan. We're the only home he knows. Get rid of me, not the cat!"

My mother wisely handled the situation by keeping me, keeping my brothers, and keeping Freedom. She hid the cat in the basement on those rare occasions when the doctor made a house call.

My nesting instincts were strong then and have not changed. My brothers kid me about how I build a nest of close friends wherever I go or live. In my junior year of college, I helped charter a new sorority on campus. My mother could not understand why I would want to belong to a sorority. She pointed out the elitism of the sorority system and the ways in which it might limit my making new friends.

I explained that I wanted to belong to a sorority. It was simply another version of the women's networks she loves so much, a community of sisters. I told her I needed a family setting to function best. I worked hard for the sorority, and it worked well for me.

The need for roots and close friends in my life is one of the reasons I can hardly wait to have a family. Recent studies by the U.S. Census Bureau show that going to college may delay marriage but seems likely to improve a woman's prospects for eventually being wed—if she wants to be and finds someone who meets her standards. That contradicts an earlier version of the study which appeared in *Newsweek* magazine and contended that a woman's chances of marriage decreased if she attended college.

As much as I want to be married and have a family one

day, it is not the driving force in my life. I doubt even a study that honestly revealed that going to college destroys marriage potential would have stopped me from getting my undergraduate degree or working for a graduate one! I have a deep belief that one day I will have it *all*: family, home and career. I can hardly wait! Then my real test will come: Will I be able to talk to my daughter about sex and make her feel good about herself? I intend to make certain that I'm not so busy listening to myself talk and getting my message across that I don't give my daughter a chance to talk, too.

I want to have children, when I'm ready and in a world that I can handle. I want to be close with my daughter and I know that will take a lot of work. I hope I'm able to do it.

Intimacy is the most important part of speaking of sex between mother and daughter. I know it's possible to establish that precious relationship: My mother and I did it.